Herbal REMEDIES

Your Complete Guide to 120 Healing Herbs & Natural Medicines

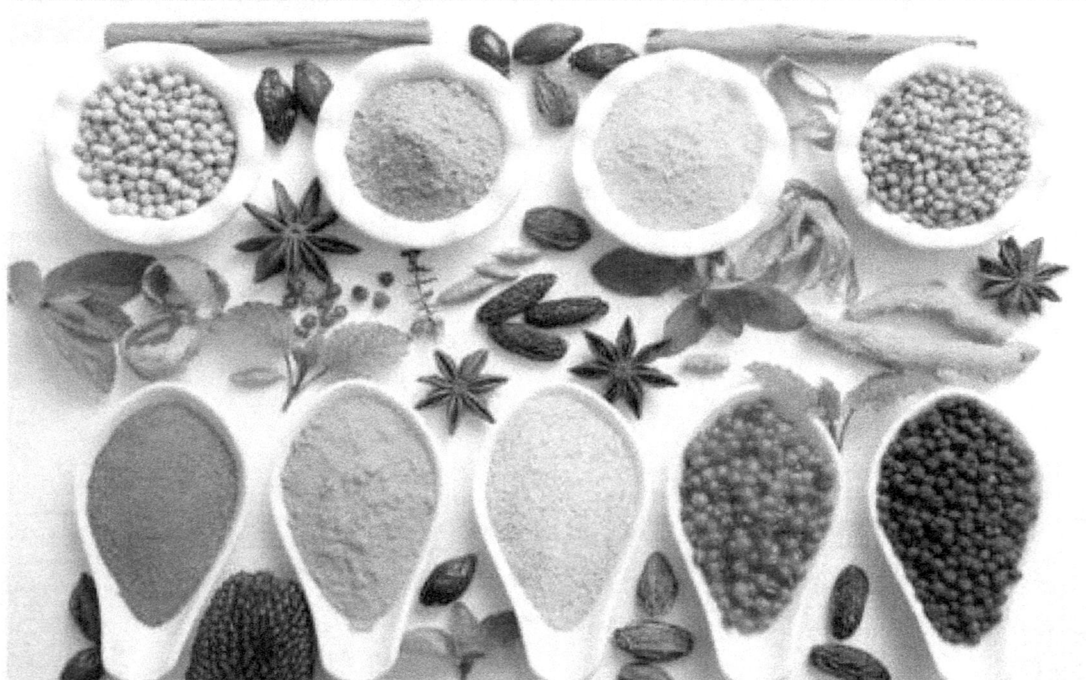

Herbal Remedies: Your Complete Guide to 120 Healing Herbs

Written by Mark Fox

Contents

Introduction

Welcome to "Herbal Remedies: Your Complete Guide to 120 Healing Herbs." In the midst of our fast-paced modern lives, there's a growing recognition of the profound wisdom encapsulated in the world of herbal remedies. This guide is your passport into the rich realm of plant-based healing, offering a comprehensive exploration of 100 herbs that have been cherished for their therapeutic properties throughout history.

Herbal remedies are more than just alternatives to conventional medicine; they represent a holistic approach to well-being, connecting us with the natural world and tapping into the innate healing powers of plants. In this guide, we embark on a journey through the lush landscapes of botanical medicine, unveiling the secrets and potential of diverse herbs that have been trusted companions on humanity's health journey for centuries.

What Awaits You in this Guide:

In-Depth Herb Profiles: Each herb featured in this guide receives a dedicated profile, providing you with a wealth of information. From the historical uses to the latest scientific findings, you'll gain a holistic understanding of the herb's healing properties.

Practical Application: Beyond knowledge, this guide equips you with practical insights on how to incorporate these herbs into your daily life. Whether you're seeking relief from common ailments or aiming to enhance your overall well-being, you'll discover user-friendly tips and recipes.

Safety Guidelines: Understanding the power of herbs comes with the responsibility of using them wisely. Throughout this guide, we emphasize safety precautions, ensuring that you approach herbal remedies with confidence and caution.

Holistic Health Approach: Herbal Remedies 101 doesn't merely focus on symptomatic relief; it delves into the holistic principles of herbalism. You'll explore herbs that support not only physical health but also mental and emotional well-being.

Cultural Wisdom: Herbs are not only healers but also bearers of cultural wisdom. Discover the historical significance, folklore, and traditional uses that have woven these herbs into the fabric of different societies.

Why Herbal Remedies Matter:

In a world inundated with synthetic medications and a sometimes overwhelming array of health options, herbal remedies offer a return to simplicity. They remind us of the intricate dance between humans and the plant kingdom—a dance that has sustained us for millennia.

As we navigate this guide, consider it your companion on a journey of self-discovery and empowerment. Whether you're a seasoned herbal enthusiast or just dipping your toes into the herbal waters, Herbal Remedies 120 is designed to be a comprehensive and accessible resource for all.

So, let the exploration begin. Open these pages, breathe in the herbal wisdom, and embark on a transformative journey with nature's apothecary. Your well-being awaits amidst the leaves, roots, and blooms of the one hundred healing herbs awaiting your discovery.

Chapter 1

Herbal Medicine

Herbal medicine, often called herbalism or phytotherapy, is the practice of utilizing plants, flower essences, and other plant-based materials for the purpose of preventing, treating, or alleviating a wide range of medical issues. So, "herbal medicine" describes the practice of using plants with therapeutic properties for the purpose of health promotion and disease prevention.

Using components found in various plant parts, including leaves, roots, stems, blossoms, and seeds, this traditional medicine has a long and storied history.

Phytotherapy, botanical medicine, and herbal medicine all refer to the practice of using plants and plant extracts for the purposes of health promotion, disease prevention, and treatment. Herbal medicine is based on time-tested concepts that have their origins in both ancient wisdom and modern scientific understanding.

Some basic ideas about herbal medicine are as follows:

1.   **A Comprehensive Approach**: Traditional herbal treatment takes a more comprehensive view of the patient, treating the full individual rather than merely their symptoms. Restoring equilibrium and promoting general health are its overarching goals.

2.   **Customized Care**: Individualized treatment plans are common among herbalists. Age, constitution, way of life, and pre-existing medical issues are among the many variables that could affect how an individual reacts to a given herb.

3.   **The Restorative Potential of Mother Nature**: Vis medicatrix naturae is another name for this theory, which states that the human body has a natural tendency to cure itself. Complementing and enhancing the body's inherent recuperative mechanisms is the goal of herbal treatment.

4.   **Health Promotion and Prevention**: Both the treatment and prevention of illness are possible with herbal therapy. A fundamental tenet is the need for health maintenance and preventative care.

5.   **Cultural Knowledge and Traditional Wisdom**: A lot of what we know about herbal therapy comes from the wisdom passed down through generations of different nations' medical traditions. Much of what is known about plant-based medicines comes from indigenous and traditional medical systems.

6.   **Utilization of Complete Plants**: To preserve the synergy of the plant's different components, herbalists frequently choose to use entire plants or extracts. It is believed that this method will increase therapeutic results while decreasing the risk of negative effects.

7.   **Reliability with Few Adverse Effects**: The goal of herbal medicine is to provide a safe and mild treatment with few unwanted side effects. Nevertheless, it is critical to acknowledge that even naturally occurring compounds can interact with one another or have negative effects in specific contexts.

8.   **Practice Based on Research and Evidence**: Herbal medicine is based on traditional knowledge, but contemporary practitioners frequently incorporate scientific studies to support and improve their techniques. Decisions about herbal treatment should be based on study findings, which is known as evidence-based herbal medicine.

9.   **Harvesting in a Sustainable and Ethical Way**: To guarantee the continued supply of medicinal herbs, herbalists frequently stress ethical and sustainable plant harvesting methods. Ethical herbal practitioners fight against habitat loss and overharvesting.

10.   **Working Together with Traditional Medical Practices**: In addition to traditional medical care, herbal remedies have their uses. Herbal therapies are often cited as part of an integrated strategy that combines them with conventional medical treatments.

If you have specific health concerns or want to combine herbal remedies with conventional therapies, it's important to see a certified healthcare expert, like a naturopath or herbalist, before using herbal medicine, even though it can be helpful.

Foundations Of Herbalism: Unveiling The Roots Of Natural Healing

Herbalism is a comprehensive approach to health and wellbeing that combines traditional knowledge, cultural practices, and an understanding of plant properties. The foundations of herbalism encompass a multitude of subjects that contribute to its complex structure.

The importance of plant Identification

Plant identification is crucial for various reasons, spanning ecological, medicinal, culinary, conservation, and safety considerations.

Here are some key points highlighting the importance of plant identification:

1. **Ecological Understanding**:

- Biodiversity Monitoring: Identifying plant species is essential for monitoring and assessing biodiversity in ecosystems. It helps scientists track changes over time, assess the health of ecosystems, and implement conservation measures.

- Ecological Research: Plant identification is fundamental to ecological research, enabling scientists to understand plant interactions, ecosystem dynamics, and the roles plants play in various environments.

2. **Medicinal and Herbal Uses:**

- Safety in Herbal Medicine: Proper plant identification is crucial for herbalists and traditional medicine practitioners to ensure the safe and effective use of medicinal plants. Incorrect identification can lead to harmful consequences and adverse reactions.

- Standardization of Herbal Products: In the herbal medicine and pharmaceutical industries, accurate plant identification is essential for standardizing herbal products and ensuring consistency in the formulation of medicines.

3. **Culinary and Edible Plants:**

- Foraging Safety: Correct plant identification is vital for foragers and wild food enthusiasts to distinguish edible plants from toxic ones. Misidentification can lead to poisoning and serious health risks.

4. **Conservation and Plant Protection**:

- Endangered Species Preservation: Plant identification plays a crucial role in identifying endangered and rare plant species. Conservation efforts rely on accurate identification to protect and preserve threatened plant populations and their habitats.

- Invasive Species Management: Identifying invasive plant species is essential for managing and controlling their spread, preventing ecological imbalances, and protecting native flora.

5. **Horticulture and Agriculture:**

- Crop Management: In agriculture, accurate plant identification is vital for managing crops, identifying pests, and implementing effective agricultural practices.

- Landscaping and Gardening: Plant identification is important for landscapers, gardeners, and horticulturists to choose suitable plants for specific environments, ensuring optimal growth and landscape design.

6. **Environmental Impact Assessment**:

- Land Use Planning: Identifying plant species is a key component of environmental impact assessments and land use planning. It helps authorities understand the potential effects of development on local ecosystems.

7. **Education and Research:**

- Botanical Studies: Proper plant identification is fundamental to botanical studies and research. It forms the basis for understanding plant taxonomy, physiology, and ecology.

- Education and Awareness: Teaching plant identification fosters environmental awareness and a deeper understanding of the natural world. It encourages responsible interaction with plants and ecosystems.

Plant identification is a foundational skill with far-reaching implications in various fields. It contributes to ecological conservation, sustainable resource use, human health and safety, and our overall understanding of the natural world. Whether for scientific research, conservation efforts, or everyday activities, the ability to identify plants is a valuable and versatile skill.

Traditional Healing Systems

Traditional healing systems are the diverse and ancient methods of treatment that have evolved over ages in various cultures. These systems frequently have their roots in the traditional knowledge and practices of individual groups.

While the terminology and methods may differ, the basic ideas are often based on a holistic approach to health, taking into account the interdependence of the body, mind, and spirit.

Here are a few notable traditional healing systems from around the world:

1. Traditional Chinese Medicine (TCM)

TCM's key components include acupuncture, herbal medicine, nutritional therapy, massage (Tui Na), and activities like Tai Chi and Qigong.

Philosophy is based on Yin and Yang concepts, the Five Elements, and the movement of Qi (energy) via the body's meridians.

Diagnosis: TCM practitioners employ methods such as pulse and tongue diagnosis to assess bodily imbalances.

2. Ayurveda:

Ayurveda, which originated in ancient India, is one of the world's oldest holistic treatment systems.

Key Components: Ayurvedic therapy consists of balancing the three doshas (Vata, Pitta, and Kapha), dietary guidelines, herbal medicines, yoga, and meditation.

Individualization: Treatments are tailored to each individual's unique constitution (Prakriti) and imbalances (Vikriti).

3. Herbalism:

Global Tradition: Herbalism is a common traditional therapeutic technique found in many cultures around the world.

Key components include the use of plants and plant-based treatments for healing. Herbalists frequently make formulations from roots, leaves, petals, and other plant components.

Herbalism frequently treats the whole individual, including lifestyle and environmental variables.

4. Native Americans' Healing Traditions:

Cultural Diversity: Native American healing practices differ by tribe, with each having its own traditions.

Ceremonies and Rituals: Healing frequently includes ceremonies, rituals, and the use of sacred plants. In medicine, men and women have important roles in these traditions.

5. Kampo Medicine:

Kampo originated in Japan and is influenced by traditional Chinese medicine.

Key Components: uses herbal treatments, acupuncture, and nutritional guidance. The diagnosis entails determining the balance of Qi and blood.

6. Unani Medicine:

Unani is derived from Greco-Arabic medicine and is widely practiced in the Middle East, South Asia, and portions of Europe.

Key Components: The emphasis is on the balance of the four humors (blood, phlegm, black bile, and yellow bile), the use of herbal medications, and lifestyle advice.

7. African Traditional Medicine:

Cultural Diversity: Healing techniques in Africa vary greatly depending on ethnicity.

Spiritual Elements: Healing frequently includes spiritual ceremonies, divination, and the use of medicinal herbs. Traditional healers may perform specific functions, such as herbalists or diviners.

8. Siddha Medicines:

Siddha medicine, a traditional therapeutic system, has its roots in India's ancient Tamil culture.

Key Components: Uses herbs, minerals, and metals to balance the three doshas (Vata, Pitta, and Kapha) and promote overall health.

9. Australian Aboriginal Medicine:

Connection to the Land: Healing techniques are inextricably linked to the land and our spiritual relationship with it.

Bush Medicine: The use of plants, also known as "bush medicine," for medicinal and therapeutic purposes.

These traditional treatment methods frequently emphasize preventive measures, lifestyle changes, and the use of natural substances to promote health and treat disease. While many traditional techniques are strongly entrenched in cultural and spiritual beliefs, they coexist with, and sometimes enhance, modern healthcare systems.

It is critical to treat these traditions with respect for cultural uniqueness and knowledge passed down through the centuries.

Chapter 2

Benefits of Natural Medicine

Herbal treatment, acupuncture, nutritional supplements, and mind-body techniques are just a few of the many techniques that fall under the umbrella of natural medicine, often known as alternative or supplementary medicine. Even if there are differences in the efficacy of natural medicine, many people value and pursue these treatments for a variety of reasons.

The following are some possible advantages to using natural medicine:

- ❖ **Holistic Approach**: Given the interdependence of the body, mind, and spirit, natural medicine frequently adopts a holistic approach to health. This method may address a condition's underlying causes and contributing elements in addition to its symptoms.

- ❖ **Emphasis on Prevention**: To preserve general health, many natural medicine methods place a strong emphasis on lifestyle changes and preventive measures. This could involve altering one's diet, exercising, practicing stress management strategies, and using herbal medicines to assist the body's inherent healing processes.

- ❖ **Diminished adverse effects**: Natural therapies may have fewer and milder adverse effects than some pharmaceutical drugs. People who are sensitive to traditional treatments or worry about their possible side effects may find this especially appealing.

- ❖ **Cultural and Traditional Wisdom**: Age-old traditional healing methods from many cultures are frequently included in natural medicine. These customs can offer a distinctive viewpoint on health and wellbeing since they are based on the cumulative knowledge of many generations.

- ❖ **Treatment Plans That Are Tailored**: A lot of practitioners of natural medicine base their treatment plans on the particular constitution, lifestyle, and medical background of each patient. Treatments that are more suited to the needs of the patient may result from this individualized care.

- ❖ **Complementary to Conventional Medicine**: Conventional medical treatments may occasionally be employed in conjunction with natural medicine. The goal of integrative medicine techniques is to maximize patient outcomes by combining the benefits of conventional and natural therapies.

- ❖ **Emphasis on Nutritional Support**: Natural medicine frequently highlights the role that nutrition plays in overall health and well-being. To address particular nutritional inadequacies, this may entail dietary suggestions, vitamin and mineral supplements, or the use of herbal medicines.

- ❖ **Mind-Body Techniques:** To encourage relaxation, lower stress levels, and improve general well-being, several natural medicine modalities—including yoga, meditation, and acupuncture—incorporate mind-body techniques.

- ❖ **Possibility of Preventing Chronic Diseases**: A lower incidence of chronic diseases has been linked to specific natural therapies and lifestyle modifications. For instance, stress reduction practices, consistent exercise, and plant-based diets may help avoid diseases like diabetes and heart disease.

- ❖ **Environmental Sustainability**: Compared to some medicines, plant-based therapies used in herbal therapy have the potential to be more environmentally friendly and sustainable. Plant species conservation is aided by ethical harvesting and cultivation techniques.

While there are benefits to natural medicine, people should approach it critically and seek the advice of licensed healthcare providers, such as naturopaths or herbalists, particularly when dealing with specific health issues or combining natural remedies with conventional treatments.

Furthermore, different people respond differently to natural medicine, so what works for one person may not work for another.

Integrating Herbal Medicine into Daily Life

A beneficial and holistic method of promoting overall health is to incorporate herbal medication into one's daily routine. The following are pragmatic suggestions for building an everyday botanical remedy regimen:

* **Acquire fundamental knowledge**:

Gain knowledge regarding common botanicals, including their characteristic attributes and potential health advantages. Recognize the vast array of applications for which botanicals can be utilized, including immune support, digestion, and relaxation.

* **Seek guidance from a phytopath or herbalist**.

Consult a proficient naturopath or herbalist for advice. Regarding your specific health concerns, personal constitution, and health objectives, they are capable of offering tailored recommendations.

* **Begin by employing basic remedies:**

Start with basic botanicals that are readily accessible. To illustrate, ginger is for immune support, chamomile is for relaxation, and peppermint is for digestion. As your familiarity with herbal remedies grows, progressively broaden your gamut.

* **Use herbal teas to supplement:**

Utilize herbal infusions as a substitute for or in addition to your customary beverages. In the morning, afternoon, or evening, savor a cup of tea selected with consideration for its therapeutic attributes. Shearing and calming properties can be found in herbal beverages.

* **Produce Infusions of Herbs:**

Herbal infusions can be integrated through the prolonged steeping of botanicals in hot water. More nutrients and compounds are extracted from the botanicals using this technique. Herbs frequently incorporated into infusions include nettle, red clover, and oat straw

❖ **Employ herbs in the kitchen**:

Cook with the assistance of culinary herbs and seasonings. Numerous botanicals possess health-promoting properties in addition to imparting flavor to food. Some examples of plants that possess antioxidant and anti-inflammatory properties are rosemary, turmeric, and garlic.

❖ **Investigate the Extracts and Tinctures of Herbs:**

Concentrated forms of herbal remedies, tinctures, and liquid extracts are available. As instructed by a qualified practitioner, add a few droplets to water or juice. For use while traveling, tinctures may be handy and portable.

Culinary Uses o f Herbs

Culinary herbs and spices play a significant role in enhancing the flavor, aroma, and nutritional value of food. Here's a detailed exploration of culinary herbs, their uses, and how to incorporate them into your cooking:

1.   Basil (Ocimum basilicum):

Flavor Profile: sweet and slightly peppery.

Culinary Uses: Fresh in salads, pesto, pasta dishes, soups, and as a topping for pizzas.

2.   Thyme (Thymus vulgaris):

Flavor Profile: earthy, slightly minty, and lemony.

Culinary Uses: Roasted meats, stews, soups, sauces, and as a seasoning for vegetables.

3.   Rosemary (Rosmarinus officinalis):

Flavor Profile: woody, pine-like, and slightly citrusy.

Culinary Uses: Roasted meats, potatoes, bread, marinades, and infused oils.

4.   Parsley (Petroselinum crispum):

Flavor Profile: Fresh, slightly peppery, and bright.

Culinary Uses: Garnish for dishes, salads, soups, sauces, and as a key ingredient in tabbouleh.

5.   Cilantro/Coriander (Coriandrum sativum):

Flavor Profile: Fresh, citrusy, and slightly spicy.

Culinary Uses: salsas, guacamole, curries, salads, and as a garnish for various international cuisines.

6.   Mint (Mentha spp.):

Flavor Profile: refreshing, sweet, and sometimes peppery.

Culinary Uses: Desserts, beverages, salads, teas, and as a garnish for savory dishes.

7.   Sage (Salvia officinalis):

Flavor Profile: earthy, slightly peppery, and savory.

Culinary Uses: Roasted meats, stuffing, pasta dishes, and as a seasoning for butter sauces.

8.   Oregano (Origanum vulgare):

Flavor Profile: robust, slightly bitter, and pungent.

Culinary Uses: Italian and Mediterranean dishes, pizza, marinades, and tomato-based sauces.

9.   Chives (Allium schoenoprasum):

Flavor Profile: mild onion flavor.

Culinary Uses: Salads, omelets, soups, and as a garnish for various dishes.

10.   Dill (Anethum graveolens):

Flavor Profile: Fresh, slightly sweet, and tangy.

Culinary Uses: Pickles, seafood dishes, salads, yogurt-based sauces, and as a garnish for potatoes.

Tips for Incorporating Culinary Herbs

1.   Fresh vs. dried:

Fresh: Use fresh herbs for maximum flavor in salads, garnishes, and dishes with short cooking times.

Dried: Dried herbs are suitable for longer-cooking dishes, marinades, and sauces.

2.   Pairing Combinations:

Classic Combos: basil and tomatoes; rosemary and roasted meats; thyme and poultry.

Experiment: Try unique combinations like mint in savory dishes or cilantro in desserts.

3.   Infused oils and vinegars:

Herb-infused Oils: Create flavored oils by infusing olive oil with rosemary, thyme, or garlic for cooking or dipping.

Herb-infused Vinegars: Infuse vinegar with herbs like tarragon, dill, or basil for dressings and marinades.

4.   Herb Butters:

Compound Butter: Mix minced herbs into softened butter for a flavorful spread on bread or to finish grilled meats.

5.   Herb Blends:

Homemade Spice Blends: Create custom spice blends by combining dried herbs like Italian seasoning, herbes de Provence, or za'atar.

6.   Herb Pesto:

Versatile Sauces: Prepare pesto with herbs like basil, parsley, or cilantro, adding nuts, garlic, and Parmesan for a versatile sauce.

7.   Herb-infused Desserts:

Sweet Treats: Experiment with adding herbs like thyme, basil, or rosemary to desserts, such as fruit salads, sorbets, or cookies.

8.   Garnishes and edible flowers:

Aesthetic Appeal: Use fresh herb sprigs, edible flowers, or microgreens as garnishes to enhance the visual appeal of dishes.

9.   Herb-infused Beverages:

Herbal Teas: Brew fresh or dried herbs like mint, chamomile, or lavender for refreshing teas.

Infused Waters: Add herbs like basil, mint, or citrus to water for a hydrating and flavorful beverage.

10.   Preserving Fresh Herbs:

Freezing: Preserve fresh herbs by freezing them in oil or water for later use in cooking.

Experimenting with culinary herbs not only enhances the flavor of your dishes but also brings a myriad of health benefits due to the rich array of phytonutrients present in these plants. Whether you have a full herb garden or a few potted plants on your windowsill, incorporating these aromatic herbs into your daily cooking can elevate your culinary experience

Herbal Infusions And Teas

Herbal infusions and teas are delightful and healthful ways to enjoy the benefits of medicinal plants. Here's an in-depth exploration of herbal infusions, their preparation methods, and some popular herbal teas:

What is an Herbal Infusion?

An herbal infusion is a concentrated liquid made by steeping herbs in hot water. It extracts the medicinal properties, flavors, and aromas of the herbs.

Preparation Method:

Ingredients: Dried or fresh herbs, hot water.

Steps:

- ❖ Boil water and pour it over the herbs.
- ❖ Allow the herbs to steep for a specific duration.
- ❖ Strain the herbs, and the resulting liquid is the herbal infusion.

Popular Herbal Infusions

1.   Chamomile Infusion

Pros: Promotes sleep, helps with digestion, and is calming.

To prepare, steep five to seven minutes' worth of dried chamomile flowers in hot water.

2.   Peppermint Infusion:

Benefits: Refreshing, aids in digestion, reduces nausea.

To prepare, steep 5 to 10 minutes in hot water with either fresh or dried peppermint leaves.

3.   Lemon Balm Infusion:

Benefits: Promotes mood, calms, and facilitates digestion.

To prepare, steep 10 minutes of fresh or dried lemon balm leaves in hot water

4.   Nettle Infusion:

Benefits: Rich in nutrients, helps with allergies, encourages detoxification.

To prepare, soak dried nettle leaves in hot water for a minimum of fifteen minutes.

5.   Rooibos Infusion:

Benefits: High in antioxidants, free of caffeine, and beneficial to the immune system.

To prepare the leaves, steep them in hot water for five to seven minutes.

Herbal Teas: A Journey into Natural Wellness

Herbal teas, also known as tisanes, are delightful and healthful infusions made from a variety of dried herbs, flowers, fruits, and spices. Embracing the goodness of nature, herbal teas offer a spectrum of flavors and potential health benefits.

Let's embark on a journey into the world of herbal teas.

1.   **Chamomile Tea:**

Flavor Profile: mild, floral, and slightly sweet.

Benefits: calming, aiding digestion, and promoting sleep.

Brewing: Steep dried chamomile flowers in hot water for 5–7 minutes. Add honey for sweetness.

2.   **Peppermint Tea:**

Flavor Profile: refreshing, minty, and invigorating.

Benefits: Digestive aid relieves nausea and soothes headaches.

Brewing: Steep fresh or dried peppermint leaves in hot water for 5–10 minutes.

3.   **Lemon Balm Tea:**

Flavor Profile: citrusy, mild, and slightly sweet.

Benefits: Calming, supporting mood, aiding digestion.

Brewing: Steep fresh or dried lemon balm leaves in hot water for 10 minutes.

4.   **Ginger Tea:**

Flavor Profile: Warm, spicy, and slightly sweet.

Benefits: anti-inflammatory, aids digestion, boosts immune system.

Brewing: Steep fresh ginger slices or dried ginger in hot water for 10–15 minutes. Add lemon for extra zest.

5.   **Turmeric Tea:**

Flavor Profile: earthy, slightly bitter, and aromatic.

Benefits: anti-inflammatory, antioxidant-rich.

Brewing: Steep ground turmeric or fresh turmeric slices in hot water. Add black pepper for enhanced absorption.

6.   **Hibiscus Tea:**

Flavor Profile: tart, fruity, and vibrant.

Benefits: Rich in antioxidants, it supports heart health.

Brewing: Steep dried hibiscus flowers in hot water for 5–10 minutes. Sweeten with honey or agave, if desired.

7.   **Lavender Tea:**

Flavor Profile: Floral, fragrant, and calming.

Benefits: relaxing, aiding sleep, anti-anxiety.

Brewing: Steep dried lavender flowers in hot water for 5–7 minutes. Enjoy before bedtime.

8.   **Nettle Tea:**

Flavor Profile: earthy, grassy, and mildly sweet.

Benefits: nutrient-rich, supports allergies, promotes detoxification.

Brewing: Steep dried nettle leaves in hot water for at least 15 minutes.

9.   **Rooibos Tea:**

Flavor Profile: Woody, sweet, and nutty.

Benefits: antioxidant-rich, caffeine-free.

Brewing: Steep rooibos leaves in hot water for 5-7 minutes. Enjoy it with or without milk.

10.   **Echinacea Tea:**

Flavor Profile: earthy, slightly bitter, and herbal.

Benefits: immune support, cold prevention.

Brewing: Steep dried echinacea root or leaves in hot water for 10–15 minutes.

11.   **Cinnamon Spice Tea:**

Flavor Profile: Warm, sweet, and aromatic.

Benefits: antioxidant-rich, anti-inflammatory.

Brewing: Combine cinnamon sticks with other spices like cloves and cardamom. Steep in hot water for 10 minutes.

12.   **Mint Medley Tea:**

A cool mixture of spearmint, peppermint, and other herbs make up the flavor profile.

Benefits: uplifting, cooling, and aiding in digestion.

Brewing: In hot water, steep a mixture of dried or fresh mint leaves for five to seven minutes.

1.   **Herbal Blends**: Try blending your own concoctions by experimenting with various herbs and spices.

2.   **Cold Infusions**: Herbal teas can be enjoyed cold by steeping them in cold water for a few hours or leaving them in the fridge overnight.

3.   **Sweeteners:** If preferred, you can use natural sweeteners like honey, agave, or maple syrup.

4.   **Citrus Zest**: Infuse your herbal teas with the zest of lemon or orange to enhance their flavors.

5.   **Insightful Drinking**: Take a moment to sip herbal tea and practice mindfulness, self-care, and relaxation.

Herbal teas provide a comprehensive approach to wellbeing in addition to stimulating the sense of taste. Accept the variety of tastes and health benefits of herbal teas as you incorporate them into your regular routines. They offer solace, sustenance, and a link to the calming wonders of the natural world.

Differences Between Herbal Infusions and Teas: Unveiling the Brew Mastery

Both teas and herbal infusions are popular drinks made from the goodness of nature, but they are not the same in terms of composition, provenance, or brewing methods. Now let's explore the differences between teas and herbal infusions:

1.   **Basic Structure:**

   1. Infusions of Herbs:

Ingredients: A range of dried herbs, flowers, fruits, and spices are used to make herbal infusions. These can include lavender, peppermint, chamomile, and other plants.

Absence of Tea Leaves: Herbal infusions do not include Camellia sinensis plant leaves, in contrast to true teas (green, black, white, and oolong).

2. Teas

Teas: Ingredients: The leaves of the Camellia sinensis plant are the source of true teas, which include green tea, black tea, white tea, and oolong tea.

Varieties: Every genuine tea variety experiences varying degrees of processing and oxidation, which contribute to unique flavors and attributes.

2.   **Content of Caffeine**:

3. Herbal Concoctions:

Caffeine-Free: Since herbal infusions are naturally caffeine-free, they are a good choice for people who are looking for a caffeine-free beverage.

4. Teas:

Caffeine Content: The amount of caffeine in real teas varies. It is generally observed that black tea contains more caffeine than green tea.

3.   **Origin of the term "tea"**:

5. Herbal Infusions:

Not Technically Tea: Herbal infusions are not, strictly speaking, teas. Traditional usage of the term "tea" describes drinks made from the Camellia sinensis plant.

6. Teas:

Origin of True Teas: The leaves of the Camellia sinensis plant are the source of true teas, which include green, black, white, and oolong teas.

4.   **Brewing Techniques**:

7. Herbal Infusions:

Preparation: Usually, dried or fresh herbs are steeped in hot water to create herbal infusions. Mint, lavender, and chamomile are common herbs.

8. Teas:

Brewing Temperatures: Depending on the variety, true teas have different brewing temperatures; for example, black tea tastes better when the water is hotter, while green tea typically needs lower temperatures.

Steeping Time: Tea leaves have precise steeping times, varying for different types and desired strengths.

5. **Flavor Profiles:**

A Range of Tastes in Herbal Infusions depending on the herbs used, herbal infusions may have a wide variety of flavors, from flowery and fruity to earthy and spicy.

Variety of Tea Flavors: True teas come in a range of flavors, including black tea's strength, oolong tea's complexity, and green tea's freshness, depending on their variety and processing techniques.

6. **Plant-Based Infusions**:

Chamomile tea is a traditional herbal infusion that is soothing.

A cool, digesting beverage to have after a meal is a peppermint infusion.

Teas: Green tea: precisely blended with subtle grassy notes and antioxidants.

The unique citrusy scent of Earl Grey Black Tea is enhanced by the addition of bergamot oil.

7. **Importance in Culture:**

Global Customs: There is a long tradition of using local herbs in traditional medicines and drinks across many cultures, which has led to the global infusion of herbal infusions.

Teas: Culture of Tea: As tea ceremonies and rituals are an essential part of everyday life in places like China, Japan, India, and England, true teas have cultural significance.

To summarize, there are differences between herbal infusions and teas in terms of ingredients, brewing methods, caffeine content, and cultural contexts, but they both enjoy the same pleasure of steeping and sipping. Either way, you can explore the flavorful and soothing world of natural brews, whether you prefer the varied world of herbal infusions or the subtle notes of true teas in particular.

Chapter 3

Common Herbs and Their Uses

In addition to adding flavor to food, these common herbs have several medical uses. Incorporating them into your regular meals or making herbal infusions can enhance your gastronomic experience and promote overall wellness.

Always check with your doctor before using any herbal supplement, but especially so if you have any preexisting issues.

1. **Ocimum basilicum, or basil, in the kitchen**: Used extensively in Mediterranean cooking due to its fragrant and sweet taste. Pasta, salads, and pesto all rely on this essential component.

   For medicinal purposes: has antioxidant and anti-inflammatory characteristics. Historically, it has served as a gentle sedative and an aid to digestion.

2. **The culinary uses of rosemary (Rosmarinus officinalis)** include enhancing the flavor of roasted meats, vegetables, and stews with its savory aroma. Mediterranean and Italian cuisines often incorporate it.

   It is well-known for its cognitive-enhancing qualities and has medicinal uses as well. Used for enhancing focus and memory in traditional medicine.

3. **Thyme,** scientifically known as Thymus vulgaris, has several culinary uses, including enhancing the flavor of roasted meats, stews, and soups. This herb is a mainstay in Mediterranean and French cooking. With antibacterial characteristics, it has medicinal uses. For the relief of respiratory symptoms and the improvement of respiratory health in general, use this.

4. **Mint (Mentha spp.)** has many culinary uses, including in drinks, sweets, and salads. Many people enjoy peppermint and spearmint.Its digestive effects are well-known among its medicinal uses. Used to alleviate headaches, nausea, and indigestion.

5. **Petroselinum crispum**, more commonly known as parsley, has many culinary uses. It freshens up salads, soups, and sauces, among other foods.For medicinal purposes:

includes minerals and vitamins. Used for its moderate diuretic and kidney-supportive traditional uses.

6. **Coriander/Cilantro (Coriandrum sativum)** : In food, it's often used in Asian, Mexican, and Middle Eastern dishes. Cinnamon leaves and coriander seeds can both be used.In medicine, It is known for being an antioxidant. Commonly used to help digestion and ease light stomach pain.

7. **Chamomile:**Also known as Matricaria chamomilla, Can be used for cooking, and also for making soothing tea. Medical Uses, It is known to calm and reduce inflammation. Used to help people relax, fall asleep, and ease stomach pain.

8. **Lavender (Lavandula angustifolia):** • Flowers are used in cooking, like in desserts and drinks that have lavender added to them.In medicine, It can calm you down and kill germs. Often found in aromatherapy and plant medicines that help with stress.

9. **Sage, or Salvia officinalis**, is used in cooking to add a savory taste to meats, soups, and stuffing. Used a lot in Thanksgiving recipes.As medicine, it has been traditionally used to ease sore throats and help digestion. Thought to help with remembering.

10. The herb **oregano, also known as Origanum** vulgare, is used in many dishes in Mediterranean and Italian cuisines. It makes pizza, pasta sauces, and cooked foods taste better.It is used in medicine because it kills germs, also used for improving the health of the lungs and the immune system.

11. **Dill, or Anethum graveolens**, gives pickles, salads, and seafood dishes a unique taste. As medicine, it has been traditionally used to ease stomach problems and make people pee more.

12. **Lemon Balm (Melissa officinalis)**: add a lemony taste to teas, salads, and desserts. In medicine, it is known to calm people down and fight viruses. Helps you relax and feel less stressed.

13. **Ginger, or Zingiber officinale**, is used in cooking to make both sweet and savory foods warmer and more flavorful. Used a lot in Asian and Indian food. For medical purposes, It is known to help with nausea and pain. Used to ease stomach pain and boost the defense system.

14. **Turmeric, or Curcuma longa**, gives curries, soups, and rice dishes a warm, earthy taste. It has antioxidant and anti-inflammatory qualities, making it useful in medicine. Used to promote overall health and the health of the joints.

15. **Urtica dioica, or nettle:** • Used in the Kitchen,the young leaves of the nettle plant are cooked and used to a variety of meals.

The abundance of vitamins and minerals makes it useful medicinally. Utilized as a natural diuretic, immune system booster, and skin health promoter.

16. **Echinacea (Echinacea purpurea):** • In the kitchen, the bitter flavor makes it an unusual ingredient for many recipes. In medicine, it is well-known for the immune-enhancing effects it has. Popular for its usage in warding against and treating the common cold.

17. **Valerian (Valeriana officinalis):** • In the kitchen, the intense, earthy scent of this herb prevents it from being used in cooking. For medicinal purposes: well-known for its relaxing and calming effects. Assists with wind**ing down and getting a better night's rest.**

18. **Fennel:** In the kitchen, it gives salads, soups, and fish a licorice flavor. Seeds and bulbs are both put to good use.

Uses in Medicine: Long-time remedy for indigestion and a general improvement in digestive health.

19. **Cayenne pepper**, scientifically known as Capsicum annuum, has many culinary applications. It is used to enhance the flavor of curries and fiery sauces, among others.

Includes capsaicin, which has analgesic effects; hence, it has medicinal uses. Internally it promotes metabolism and topically it alleviates discomfort.

20. **Garlic (Allium sativum):** • In the kitchen, it is a flavor enhancer and a culinary mainstay in many different cuisines. Commonly utilized when finely chopped or crushed.In medicine, it has antibacterial and antifungal effects. Historically, it has been utilized to promote heart health and strengthen the immune system.

21. **Arnica (Arnica montana):** • In the Kitchen: Not recommended for use in the kitchen because of the possibility of toxicity.
Medicinal Uses: Applying the herb topically helps alleviate inflammation, muscle pain, and bruising.

22. **Calendula (Calendula officinalis):** • In the kitchen, the flower petals are employed in soups, salads, and as a decorative accent. Brings out a subtle, peppery taste. In the medical field, it has a reputation for reducing inflammation and calming the skin. Use on skin disorders and wounds to promote healing.

23. **Catnip, or Nepeta cataria:** In the kitchen, the leaves can be used to make tea and salads, but cat games are what they're best known for.

• Medical Uses: It has been used for a long time to calm the nervous system. It is often added to herbal teas to help people rest.

24. **Saw palmetto, or Serenoa repens**, is a plant that is not usually used in cooking.

• As a medicine, it has traditionally been used to help men keep their prostates healthy. It is often found in herbal products.

25. **St. John's Wort (Hypericum perforatum):** Not used in cooking because it might mix badly with some medicines.

• Medical Uses: It is thought to have antidepressant qualities. Herbal medicine used to treat mild to heavy depression.

26. **Holy Basil (Ocimum sanctum),** it is used in drinks and other foods. It is also called Tulsi in Ayurvedic thought.

• Medical Uses: This adaptogenic plant is used to fight stress and improve health in general.

27. **Passionflower (Passiflora incarnata):** • Leaves can be used to make tea. The fruit is sometimes used in cooking scenarios.

Uses in medicine: It is known to calm and sleepy people. Used to help people feel less anxious and more relaxed.

28. **Licorice Root (Glycyrrhiza glabra):** • In cooking, it is used to add sweetness to teas and sweets.

• Medical Uses: It is known to reduce inflammation and soothe the skin. Used to help with breathing and digestion.

29. **Ashwagandha (Withania somnifera)** is not usually used in foods.

• Medicinal Uses: This adaptogenic herb is used to fight stress, boost energy, and support general health.

30. The **astragalus plant (Astragalus membranaceus)**:

• Uses in cooking: In traditional Chinese cooking, roots are used in soups and stews.

• Medical Uses: It is known to boost the defense system and help the body adapt. Helps keep your nervous system healthy in general.

31. Ginkgo Biloba (Ginkgo biloba): Not used in situations related to cooking.

• Medicinal Uses: Renowned for improving brain function. Supports memory and brain function.

32. As for **black cohosh (Actaea racemosa)**, it's not used in cooking.

Traditional uses include treating menopause symptoms like hot flashes and mood swings.

33. **Burdock (Arctium lappa)**: The root is used in soups and stir-fries.

• Medical Uses: Recognized for its ability to clean the body. Useful for keeping skin healthy and aiding in cleansing.

34. For food, **hawthorn (Crataegus spp.**) berries can be used in jams and syrups.

• Medical Uses: is known to be good for the heart. Used to help keep the heart healthy and the blood flowing normally.

35. **Milk Thistle (Silybum marianum)**: • Medicinal Uses: The seeds can be ground up and added to food, but the plant is mostly used for its health benefits.

Medicinal Uses: It is known to protect the liver. Supports liver health and cleansing.

36. **Red Clover (Trifolium pratense)**: • Flowers can be used in drinks and salads.

Medicinal Uses: Traditionally used to improve the health of women. Supports the balance of hormones and skin problems.

37. **Yellow Dock (Rumex crispus)**: • Leaves can be used in salads, but it is mostly used for their healing qualities.

• Medical Uses: It is known to be a weak laxative and support detoxification. Utilized to improve gut health.

38. **Red Yam (Dioscorea villosa)**:

• Doesn't usually get used in cooking.

Medicinal Uses: Traditionally used to improve the health of women. Supports biological balance and eases the pain of menstruation.

39. **Oregon Grape Root (Mahonia aquifolium):**

•   Culinary Uses: Berries can be used in jams, but it is primarily used for its medicinal properties.

•   Medicinal Uses: Known for its antimicrobial properties. Used to support immune health and skin conditions.

40. **Bilberry (Vaccinium myrtillus):**

•Culinary Uses: Berries can be used in jams and desserts.

•Medicinal Uses: Known for its antioxidant properties. Used to support vision and overall eye health.

•These additional herbs offer a diverse range of flavors and medicinal properties. Whether incorporated into culinary creations or used in herbal remedies, these herbs contribute to a holistic approach to well-being. As always, it's essential to consult with a healthcare professional, especially if you have specific health concerns or conditions.

41. **Brahmi (Bacopa monnieri):**

•Culinary Uses: Not commonly used in culinary applications.

•Medicinal Uses: Known for its cognitive-enhancing properties. Used to support memory and concentration.

42. **Gotu Kola (Centella asiatica):**

•Culinary Uses: Leaves can be used in salads but is more commonly used in traditional medicine.

•Medicinal Uses: Known for its adaptogenic properties. Used to support cognitive function and overall well-being.

43. **Devil's Claw (Harpagophytum procumbens):**

•Culinary Uses: Not used in culinary applications.

•Medicinal Uses: Known for its anti-inflammatory properties. Traditionally used to alleviate joint pain and discomfort.

44. Kava Kava (Piper methysticum):

•Culinary Uses: Roots are used to prepare traditional beverages in the South Pacific but not commonly used in other cuisines.

•Medicinal Uses: Known for its relaxing and anxiety-reducing properties. Used in traditional ceremonies for its calming effects.

45. Rhodiola (Rhodiola rosea):

•Culinary Uses: Not commonly used in culinary applications.

•Medicinal Uses: Known for its adaptogenic properties. Used to combat stress, enhance endurance, and support mental clarity.

46. Borage (Borago officinalis):

•Culinary Uses: Flowers and leaves can be used in salads and beverages.

•Medicinal Uses: Known for its anti-inflammatory properties. Traditionally used to support skin health and reduce stress.

47. Evening Primrose (Oenothera biennis):

•Culinary Uses: Seeds can be used in salads and dishes, but it is primarily used for its oil.

•Medicinal Uses: Known for its gamma-linolenic acid (GLA) content. Used to support hormonal balance and skin conditions.

48. Dong Quai (Angelica sinensis): • Rarely used in cooking.

• Medical Uses: Utilized in Chinese medicine for women's health, menstrual relief, and hormone balance.

49. The Horehound (Marrubium vulgare) plant has culinary uses such as teas and candies due to its leaves.

• Utilized medicinally for expectorant qualities. Used to relieve respiratory problems and improve lung function.

50. **Witch Hazel** (Hamamelis virginiana): • No culinary use.

• Utilized medicinally for its astringent and anti-inflammatory effects. Externally applied for skin problems and natural toner.

51. **Chaste Tree (Vitex agnus-castus)**: • Rarely used in cooking.

• Medicinal Uses: Traditionally used for PMS relief, hormone balancing, and women's health support.

52. **Butterbur (Petasites hybridus)**: • Historically used in cooking, but can be hazardous when uncooked.

• It has anti-inflammatory qualities and is used medicinally. Reduces migraines and improves respiratory health.

53. **Juniper (Juniperus communis)**: • Culinary Uses: Berries are commonly used as a spice in European cuisine.

• It has diuretic qualities and is used medicinally. Traditionally used for digestion and kidney health.

54. **Yarrow (Achillea millefolium)**: • Uses: Flowers and leaves in salads and mild spices.

• Utilized medicinally for its anti-inflammatory and astringent qualities. Promotes wound healing and intestinal relief.

55. **Celandine (Chelidonium majus)**:

• Culinary Uses: Rarely utilized in cooking.

• Medical Uses: Known for antibacterial capabilities. Used for liver and intestinal health.

56. **Mullein (Verbascum thapsus):** • Historically used in teas, but not widely employed in modern cooking.

• Medicinal Uses: Effective in calming the respiratory system. Promotes lung health and reduces respiratory pain.

57. **Meadowsweet (Filipendula ulmaria):** • The flowers and leaves can be used in teas and light flavorings.

• Medical Benefits: Anti-inflammatory and digestive qualities. Used to relieve intestinal discomfort and improve digestion.

58. **Blue Vervain (Verbena hastata)**: • Teas include leaves and blossoms, but not usually used in cooking.

• Medical Benefits: Calming and nervine qualities. Reduces stress and tension.

59. Skullcap (Scutellaria lateriflora): • Rarely used in cooking.

• Medical Benefits: Calming and nervine qualities. Helps relax and support the neurological system.

60. Cleavers (Galium aparine): • Use young leaves and stems in salads and teas.

• It has diuretic qualities and is used medicinally. Used for lymphatic health and detoxification.

61. Mugwort (Artemisia vulgaris): • Culinary purposes: Use leaves sparingly in dishes and as a seasoning element in Asian cuisines.

• Medicinal Uses: Known for digestive and antibacterial effects. Used to relieve intestinal discomfort and improve gut health.

62. Bee Balm (Monarda didyma): • Use its flowers and leaves in teas and salads. Also known as Oswego tea in Native American cuisine. • It has antibacterial qualities for medicinal purposes. Used to improve digestion and health.

63. Levisticum officinale -- Lovage

• Use leaves and stems in soups, stews, and salads for a celery-like flavor.

• Medical Uses: Traditionally for digestive assistance. Contains antioxidants.

64.The **Wood Betony (Stachys officinalis)** has limited culinary uses, but its leaves and blossoms can be used in teas.

• Medical Benefits: Calming and nervine qualities. Reduces stress and tension.

65. Comfrey (Symphytum officinale): • Historically used in teas and soups, internal usage is unclear due to liver damage.

• Medical Uses: Externally for wound healing and poultice. Contains tissue-repairing allantoin.

66. Joe-Pye Weed (Eutrochium purpureum): • Rarely used in cooking.

• Medicinal Uses: Traditionally used for diuretic qualities. Supports kidney and urinary tract health.

67.The **flower of Hibiscus (Hibiscus sabdariffa**) is utilized in culinary recipes and as a bright herbal tea.

• Medical Uses: Offers antioxidant benefits. A pleasant drink and cardiovascular health aid.

68. **Chicory (Cichorium intybus**): • Uses: Leaves and roots in salads, prepared foods, and replacing coffee.

• Medical Uses: Traditionally for digestive assistance. Contains prebiotic inulin.

69. **Pennyroyal (Mentha pulegium**): • Historically used in culinary dishes and beverages, avoid internal usage due to poisonous pulegone component.

• Medical Applications: Traditionally used for insect repellence and skin treatment.

70. In South America, **Yerba Mate (Ilex paraguariensis**) is used to make a stimulating herbal drink.

• It has stimulating qualities and is used medicinally. Used to boost focus and alertness.

71. **Red Root (Ceanothus americanus):**

•Culinary Uses: Not commonly used in culinary applications.

•Medicinal Uses: Traditionally used for its lymphatic and immune-supporting properties. Used to promote lymphatic drainage.

72. **Tansy (Tanacetum vulgare):**

•Culinary Uses: Historically used in small quantities in certain culinary dishes. Internal use is not recommended due to its high thujone content, which can be toxic.

•Medicinal Uses: Traditionally used for digestive support and as an external remedy for skin conditions.

73. **Wormwood (Artemisia absinthium):**

•Culinary Uses: Historically used in small quantities in certain alcoholic beverages, such as absinthe. Internal use is not recommended due to its high thujone content, which can be toxic.

•Medicinal Uses: Traditionally used for digestive support and as an external remedy for skin conditions.

74. Marshmallow (Althaea officinalis):

•Culinary Uses: Roots and leaves can be used in teas and as a thickening agent in certain culinary dishes.

•Medicinal Uses: Known for its mucilaginous properties. Used to soothe and coat the respiratory and digestive tract.

75. Angelica (Angelica archangelica):

•Culinary Uses: Stems and seeds can be used in culinary dishes, particularly in Scandinavian cuisine.

•Medicinal Uses: Traditionally used for digestive support and as an expectorant. Contains compounds believed to have anti-inflammatory effects.

76. Elecampane (Inula helenium):

•Culinary Uses: Historically used in certain culinary dishes, but not commonly used today.

•Medicinal Uses: Traditionally used for respiratory support. Contains compounds believed to have expectorant and antimicrobial properties.

77. Coltsfoot (Tussilago farfara):

•Culinary Uses: Historically used in certain culinary dishes, but not commonly used today.

•Medicinal Uses: Traditionally used for respiratory support. Contains compounds believed to have expectorant and anti-inflammatory properties.

78. Bistort (Polygonum bistorta):

•Culinary Uses: Historically used in certain culinary dishes, but not commonly used today.

•Medicinal Uses: Traditionally used for digestive support. Contains compounds believed to have astringent properties.

79. Artemisia dracunculus (tarragon):

• Culinary Uses: Leaves impart an anise-like flavor to recipes.

• Medicinal Uses: Historically for digestive assistance. Includes somewhat sedative chemicals.

80. The **Lemon Verbena (Aloysia citrodora)** leaves offer a lemony flavor to drinks, sweets, and culinary items

• Medical Uses: Well-known for soothing and digestive benefits. Reduces stomach discomfort and relaxes.

81. **Costmary (Tanacetum balsamita):** • Historically used in teas and foods, current usage is rare.

• Medical Uses: Traditionally for digestive assistance. Has astringent chemicals.

82. The leaves of **Chervil (Anthriscus cerefolium)** are used in French cuisine to impart a slight anise-like flavor to meals.

• Medicinal Uses: Historically for digestive assistance. May have minor diuretic properties.

83. **Southernwood (Artemisia abrotanum):** • Historically used in teas and dishes, but not often used today.

• Medical Uses: Traditionally for digestive assistance. Has weak insect-repelling chemicals.

84. **Lovage (Levisticum officinale):** • Adds celery-like flavor to soups, stews, and salads.

• Medical Uses: Traditionally for digestive assistance. Contains antioxidants.

85. **Chickweed (Stellaria media):** • Use foliage in salads and meals.

• Medical Benefits: Anti-inflammatory and demulcent qualities. Used for respiratory support and skin disorders.

86. **Basil Sweet (Ocimum basilicum):** • Uses: Leaves are commonly used in Italian cuisine.

• Medical Benefits: Anti-inflammatory and antioxidant capabilities. Traditional digestive aid and light sedative.

87. **Borage (Borago officinalis)** has flowers and leaves that can be utilized in salads and beverages.

• It has anti-inflammatory qualities and is used medicinally. Traditionally used for stress reduction and skin health.

88. **Centaury (Centaurium erythraea):** • Historically used in teas and cuisines, but not often used anymore.

• Medical Uses: Traditionally for digestive assistance. Ingredients may be bitter tonic.

89. **Cress (Lepidium sativum):** • Use leaves and stems in salads and sandwiches.

• Contains vitamins and minerals for medicinal purposes. Long used for its mild expectorant effects.

90. Alfalfa (Medicago sativa): Used as a nutritive herb to support overall health and as a mild diuretic.

91. **Angelica (Angelica archangelica):** Used to support digestion, relieve gas and bloating, and as a uterine tonic for menstrual irregularities.

92. **Burdock (Arctium lappa):** Used as a blood purifier, diuretic, and to support skin health in conditions such as eczema and acne.

93. **Catnip (Nepeta cataria):** Known for its calming effects, catnip is used to relieve anxiety, insomnia, and digestive discomfort.

94. **Cayenne (Capsicum annuum):** Used as a culinary spice and in herbal medicine for its circulatory stimulant properties to improve digestion and relieve pain.

95. **Chaste Tree (Vitex agnus-castus):** Used to regulate hormone levels, alleviate symptoms of PMS and menopause, and support reproductive health.

96. **Dong Quai (Angelica sinensis):** Used in traditional Chinese medicine to support women's health, regulate menstrual cycles, and alleviate menopausal symptoms.

97. **Fennel (Foeniculum vulgare):** Used to relieve gas, bloating, and digestive discomfort, and to support lactation in breastfeeding women.

98. **Feverfew (Tanacetum parthenium):** Used to prevent and alleviate migraines, reduce fever, and relieve menstrual cramps.

99. **Gentian (Gentiana lutea):** Used as a bitter tonic to stimulate digestion and appetite, and to relieve gas and bloating.

100. **Goldenseal (Hydrastis canadensis):** Known for its antimicrobial properties, goldenseal is used to support immune function and aid digestion.

101. **Hops (Humulus lupulus):** Used to promote relaxation, relieve anxiety and insomnia, and support digestion.

102. **Horsetail (Equisetum arvense):** Used to support bone health, strengthen hair and nails, and as a mild diuretic.

103. **Juniper (Juniperus communis**): Used as a diuretic to support kidney health, promote detoxification, and relieve digestive discomfort.

104. **Kava (Piper methysticum**): Known for its calming effects, kava is used to relieve anxiety, promote relaxation, and improve sleep.

105**. Lemon Balm (Melissa officinalis**): Used to relieve anxiety, promote relaxation, and support digestive health.

106. **Marshmallow (Althaea officinalis):** Known for its demulcent properties, marshmallow is used to soothe sore throats, coughs, and digestive irritation.

107. **Mullein (Verbascum thapsus):** Used as an expectorant to relieve coughs, congestion, and respiratory infections.

108. **Red Clover (Trifolium pratense**): Used as a blood purifier, diuretic, and to support skin health in conditions such as eczema and psoriasis.

109**. Rhodiola (Rhodiola rosea):** Used as an adaptogen to reduce stress, improve energy levels, and support mental and physical performance.

110. **Saw Palmetto (Serenoa repens**): Used to support prostate health, relieve urinary symptoms, and promote hair growth in men.

111. **Skullcap (Scutellaria lateriflora**): Known for its calming effects, skullcap is used to relieve anxiety, nervous tension, and insomnia.

112**. Slippery Elm (Ulmus rubra**): Known for its demulcent properties, slippery elm is used to soothe sore throats, coughs, and digestive irritation.

113. **Stinging Nettle (Urtica dioica**): Used as a nutritive herb to support overall health, as a diuretic, and to relieve allergies and arthritis.

114**. Vervain (Verbena officinalis**): Used to promote relaxation, relieve anxiety, and support digestive health.

115. **White Willow Bark (Salix alba**): Known for its analgesic and anti-inflammatory properties, white willow bark is used to relieve pain, inflammation, and fever.

116. **Wild Yam (Dioscorea villosa)**: Used to support women's health, balance hormone levels, and alleviate menstrual and menopausal symptoms.

117. **Witch Hazel (Hamamelis virginiana)**: Used topically as an astringent to tone and tighten the skin, relieve inflammation, and promote wound healing.

118. **Yarrow (Achillea millefolium)**: Used topically for its hemostatic properties to stop bleeding and promote wound healing, and internally to reduce fever and support digestion.

119. **Yellow Dock (Rumex crispus)**: Used as a blood purifier, mild laxative, and to support liver and digestive health.

120. **Goldenseal (Hydrastis canadensis)**: Known for its antimicrobial properties, goldenseal is used to support immune function and aid digestion

Chapter 4

Medical Botany and Pharmacognosy

Medical botany and pharmacognosy are two closely related fields that focus on the study of plants in the context of medicine, drug discovery, and the development of pharmaceutical products. Both disciplines involve the identification, characterization, and utilization of plant-derived substances for therapeutic purposes.

- Medical Botany:

Definition: Medical botany is the branch of botany that specifically deals with the study of plants used in traditional medicine as well as their potential pharmacological properties.

Objectives:

- Identification and classification of plants with medicinal properties.
- Documentation of traditional uses of plants in different cultures.
- Exploration of plant compounds for their potential pharmaceutical applications.

Methods:

- Field surveys were conducted to identify and collect medicinal plants.
- Taxonomic studies are used to classify and catalog plant species.
- Ethnobotanical research is used to document traditional knowledge and uses.

Applications:

- Provides a scientific basis for the integration of traditional medicine into modern healthcare.
- Supports the identification of potential sources for novel drug discovery.
- Contributes to the conservation of medicinal plant species.

- **Pharmacognosy**:

Definition: Pharmacognosy is the science that studies the physical, chemical, biochemical, and biological properties of drugs, drug substances, or potential pharmaceutical agents obtained from natural sources, particularly plants.

Objectives:

- Identification and standardization of plant-derived drugs.
- Isolation and characterization of bioactive compounds from natural sources.
- Evaluation of the pharmacological activities of natural products.

Methods:

- Extraction and isolation techniques to obtain bioactive compounds.
- Chromatographic and spectroscopic methods for compound identification.
- Bioassays and pharmacological studies to assess therapeutic potential.

Applications:

- Contributes to the development of new pharmaceuticals from natural sources.
- Provides quality control measures for herbal medicines and plant-based products.
- Investigates the pharmacological mechanisms of action of plant-derived compounds.

Medical botany focuses on the identification and documentation of plants used in traditional medicine, while pharmacognosy delves deeper into the chemical and pharmacological aspects of these plants, with the aim of discovering and developing novel therapeutic agents.

Both fields play crucial roles in understanding the relationship between plants and medicine, contributing to drug discovery, and ensuring the safety and efficacy of plant-based pharmaceuticals. Integrating traditional knowledge with modern scientific methods in these disciplines can lead to the development of valuable and evidence-based medicinal product.

Nourishing the Body, Mind, and Spirit

A healing diet is a detailed nutritional regimen that focuses on eating foods rich in nutrients to support the body's innate healing mechanisms. It considers both physical health and mental and emotional well-being. This is an in-depth analysis of therapeutic diets, including visual aids and key concepts.

Principles of Healing Diets

1. Whole, Nutrient-Dense Foods:

It is important to eat whole foods that are high in vitamins, minerals, and antioxidants. Just as an example: Fruits, nuts, vegetables, whole grains, and lean protein should all be part of your diet.

Whole foods that have been minimally processed and are high in nutrients have many important nutrients like vitamins, minerals, fiber, and antioxidants. These foods are good for your health and well-being in general.

Full, nutrient-dense foods are described below:

- ❖ Some leafy greens that are good for you are spinach, collard greens, kale, and Swiss chard. They are high in minerals like calcium and iron, as well as vitamins A, C, and K.
- ❖ Broccoli, tomatoes, carrots, bell peppers, and other colorful vegetables are full of vitamins and antioxidants.
- ❖ Berries: Raspberries, blueberries, and strawberries are all high in fiber, vitamins, and antioxidants for a fruit.
- ❖ Citrus fruits, like oranges, grapefruits, and lemons, are full of vitamin C and other good things for you.
- ❖ Bananas: These fruits are high in potassium and full of minerals and vitamins that your body needs. They also give you energy.

2. **Whole Grains:**
   - ❖ Quinoa is a whole protein since it contains fiber, iron, and magnesium.
   - ❖ The soluble fiber in oats increases energy and is good for your heart.
   - ❖ Oatmeal's soluble fiber content boosts energy and supports heart health.

3. **Lean Proteins:**
   - ❖ The amino acid profile of chicken breast makes it a great lean protein source.
   - ❖ Salmon, mackerel, trout, and other fatty fish are good for your heart because they contain omega-3 fatty acids.
   - ❖ Beans, chickpeas, lentils, and lentils—which are rich in fiber—are legumes.
   - ❖ Avocado is an excellent source of monounsaturated lipids, vitamins E and K, and folate.

4. **Nuts and seeds**, such as flaxseeds, almonds, walnuts, and chia seeds, are rich in protein, vitamins, and healthful fats.
   - ❖ Antioxidants and monounsaturated lipids are abundant in extra virgin olive oil, which is an integral part of the Mediterranean diet.

5. **Substitutes for dairy**:
   - ❖ Greek yogurt is an excellent source of bacteria and protein, both of which are advantageous for digestive health.
   - ❖ Vitamin D, protein, and calcium are all present in cheese. Select varieties that contain less sodium.
   - ❖ Plant-Based Substitutes Almond milk, soy milk, and oat milk all contain calcium and vitamin D.

6. **Spices and Herbs:**
   - ❖ Curcumin, which is present in turmeric, is recognized for its anti-inflammatory attributes.
   - ❖ Cinnamon: May aid in blood sugar regulation and impart flavor.

- ❖ Garlic is recognized for its potential to provide cardiovascular support, among other health benefits.

It is critical for one's overall wellbeing to maintain adequate hydration. Without added carbohydrates or calories, water is the optimal choice for maintaining hydration.

Chapter 5

Herbal Remedies For Diseases

Herbal medicines should be carefully studied and used cautiously due to the potential for unfavorable interactions with pharmaceuticals or contraindications. Herbal treatments can provoke various reactions in people. It is crucial to regularly seek advice from a healthcare expert, especially whether pregnant, breastfeeding, or dealing with pre-existing health issues.

Historically, herbal treatments have been used to cure various health ailments and improve overall well-being. It is crucial to recognize that while some herbal medicines may offer comfort or aid, they should not be viewed as a substitute for professional medical advice or treatment. Consult a healthcare practitioner before incorporating herbal remedies into your everyday medical routine.

These herbal treatments have a lengthy history of being used to address particular health conditions:

1. **Chamomile for Digestive Issues**: Chamomile, extracted from the flowers of the Asteraceae family, is a renowned herb with a long history of potential health advantages. Chamomile is commonly linked to relaxing and has a reputation for its effectiveness in treating digestive problems.

Here are further specifics regarding chamomile and its possible impacts on digestive well-being:

Advantages: Soothing and anti-inflammatory.

Utilizations: Insomnia, anxiety, gastrointestinal problems.

Symptoms: Indigestion, bloating, and gastrointestinal discomfort.

Preparation: Brew chamomile tea using dried chamomile flowers.

Active Compounds:

- ❖ Chamazulene: This compound has anti-inflammatory properties and contributes to the blue color of chamomile oil.

❖ Apigenin: A flavonoid found in chamomile, apigenin is known for its anti-inflammatory and antioxidant effects.

❖ Bisabolol: This compound has anti-inflammatory and anti-irritant properties, contributing to chamomile's soothing effects.

Digestive Benefits:

Chamomile is thought to possess antispasmodic properties that aid in relaxing smooth muscles in the gastrointestinal tract. This could alleviate cramping and discomfort.

Chamazulene and apigenin compounds have anti-inflammatory properties that might alleviate inflammation in the digestive system, perhaps offering relief for illnesses such as gastritis.

• Gas Relief for Indigestion and Gas:

Chamomile tea is frequently employed to mitigate gas and bloating symptoms, potentially attributable to its carminative attributes which facilitate gas elimination from the digestive tract.Chamomile aid in gastric soothing and the alleviation of indigestion symptoms.

• Irritable Bowel Syndrome (IBS):

While individual responses may differ, some individuals with irritable bowel syndrome (IBS) find alleviation from symptoms including abdominal pain and bloating by utilizing chamomile.

Consumption Methods

A common and beloved way to enjoy chamomile is in a cup of hot tea. Infusing dried chamomile flowers in hot water unleashes its therapeutic components. The medicinal properties of dried chamomile flowers can be extracted by steeping them in hot water.

If you'd rather not drink tea but still want a strong source of chamomile, you can find chamomile supplements in a variety of formats, such as capsules or tinctures.

• Considerations and Safety: Generally Safe: Most people don't have any problems with consuming moderate doses of chamomile. Nonetheless, ragweed and other members of the Asteraceae family can trigger severe allergic reactions in certain people.

Overconsumption of chamomile during pregnancy may raise the chance of miscarriage, so it is important for pregnant women to talk to their doctor before using the herb.

•In the kitchen: Chamomile adds a subtle, flowery flavor to a variety of foods and isn't just reserved for tea.Chamomile is utilized in culinary applications beyond tea, adding a subtle flowery taste to specific meals.

Overconsumption of chamomile during pregnancy may raise the chance of miscarriage, so it is important for pregnant women to talk to their doctor before using the herb.

Chamomile is generally safe for most individuals when ingested in moderate quantities. Individuals with sensitivities to plants in the Asteraceae family, such as ragweed, may develop allergic responses.

2. Turmeric

The Curcuma longa plant, originally from Southeast Asia, is the source of turmeric, a vibrantly colored spice. For ages, it has been a staple in Indian and Southeast Asian food and traditional medicine. Many of turmeric's purported health advantages are attributable to a chemical called curcumin.

•Active Compound:

Curcumin: Turmeric's principal bioactive ingredient gives it its brilliant color. Curcumin is antioxidant and anti-inflammatory.

• Anti-Inflammatory Effects:

Nuclear factor-kappa B and other inflammatory molecules are inhibited by curcumin. Doing so may minimize molecular inflammation.

Cytokine Modulation: Curcumin may alter cytokine production, which influences inflammation.

•Conditions with Inflammation:

Arthritis: Patients suffering from rheumatoid arthritis or osteoarthritis may find relief from joint stiffness and discomfort by taking curcumin, according to studies.

In inflammatory bowel diseases (IBD), curcumin's anti-inflammatory actions have demonstrated encouraging results in preclinical investigations. These illnesses include Crohn's disease and ulcerative colitis.

Although studies are still in their early stages, curcumin shows promise as a treatment for inflammation in a variety of inflammatory diseases and conditions, including diabetes, neurological disorders, cardiovascular disease, and others.

• Function as an Antioxidant:

Damage to Cells and Inflammation-Inducing Free Radicals: Curcumin's Antioxidant Capacity Assists In Neutralizing These Radicals.

Modalities of Intake:

One popular use of turmeric powder in cooking is to spice up foods. Having said that, turmeric powder does not contain a particularly high concentration of curcumin.

To get a higher concentration of the active ingredient, you can take a supplement containing curcumin or an extract of the spice.

Obstacles to Bioavailability:

Curcumin is not readily absorbed by the body due to its limited bioavailability. The piperine in black pepper, when combined with it, can increase its absorption.

• Considerations and Safety: Turmeric and curcumin, at modest doses, are thought to be safe for the majority of individuals. Some people may experience gastrointestinal problems with high doses or prolonged use, though.

Curcumin has the potential to interact with other pharmaceuticals, particularly those that thin the blood. Talk to your doctor if you are on any kind of medicine.

• In the kitchen, turmeric is an essential component of curry powders and a versatile spice that enhances the taste and appearance of many different foods.

Talk to your doctor before taking any supplements containing curcumin or turmeric for any health issues, particularly if you are already on any drugs or have any preexisting illnesses.

Supplements containing turmeric or curcumin should not be taken in place of prescription drugs without first consulting a doctor.

3. Echinacea

Echinacea is a widely used herbal medicine for immune support. Echinacea is obtained from the purple coneflower plants belonging to the Echinacea genus. Different species such as Echinacea purpurea, Echinacea angustifolia, and Echinacea pallida are utilized for their therapeutic properties. Here are further specifics regarding Echinacea and its possible impact on immune support.

Echinacea for Immune Support:

It is claimed that echinacea improves the immune system by enhancing natural killer and macrophage activity. Supports the immunological system generally.

According to study, echinacea may have antiviral characteristics that reduce cold severity and duration.

People use echinacea to treat or prevent cold, flu and other upper respiratory infections during season, it is often taken as a supplement to boost immunity.

•You can consume echinacea pills or capsules.

•The liquid extracts of echinacea can be combined with water or other liquids.

Echinacea tea is made by soaking dried flowers, leaves, or roots in boiling water.

Conditions: Common colds, influenza, and immune system enhancement.

Preparation: Use Echinacea tea or capsules at the beginning of cold symptoms.

• Active Ingredients:

Alkamides are thought to possess immune-stimulating qualities and play a role in Echinacea's possible benefits.

Echinacea includes polyphenols that have antioxidant qualities, which can help fight oxidative stress and promote general health.

Polysaccharides are intricate carbohydrates present in Echinacea that might play a role in its immunomodulatory actions.

Safety and Things to Think About Echinacea

Most people think that echinacea is safe to use for a short time. Long-term use, on the other hand, may make it less useful.

Possible Allergic responses: Some people may be allergic to echinacea, and allergic responses can happen. People who are allergic to plants in the family Asteraceae should be careful.

Drug interactions: Echinacea may not work well with some medicines, especially those that weaken the immune system. If you are taking medications, you should talk to a medical expert.

• **Uses in cooking:** Echinacea is used mostly in the form of supplements or teas for medical reasons, so it isn't often used in cooking.

It's best to talk to a doctor before taking Echinacea or any other herbal product to boost your immune system. This is especially important if you already have a health problem or are on medication. Without proper medical guidance, herbal supplements should not be used instead of prescription drugs.

4. Peppermint for Irritable Bowel Syndrome (IBS):

Peppermint (Mentha x piperita) is a well-known herb that smells and tastes great. Peppermint oil, in particular, has been studied for its possible benefits in controlling symptoms of irritable bowel syndrome (IBS). It has been used for many health reasons in the past.

 Here are some more facts about peppermint and how it can help with IBS:

•Calming and good for digestion.

•Helps with stomachaches, sickness, and headaches.

Compounds that work:

- ❖ Menthol, the main chemical that makes peppermint work, has been shown to relax smooth muscles.
- ❖ Menthone is another chemical that is found in peppermint oil and helps give it its unique taste and smell.
- ❖ Terpenes: Peppermint has terpenes in it. Terpenes are aromatic organic molecules that might have health benefits.

How it affects Irritable Bowel Syndrome (IBS):

- ❖ **Relaxing Smooth Muscles**: Peppermint oil is thought to have antispasmodic properties that help calm the muscles in the digestive system. This may help ease the pain and cramping in the stomach that come with IBS.
- ❖ **Relieving Pain**: Letting go of tight muscles may help ease the pain and soreness in the abdomen.

Studies in the clinic:

- ❖ **Lessening the symptoms of IBS:** Some clinical studies have shown that peppermint oil may help ease the symptoms of IBS, like abdominal pain, bloating, and gas, especially when taken in enteric-coated pills that keep the oil from breaking down in the stomach.
- ❖ Irritable Bowel Syndrome with Diarrhea (IBS-D): Peppermint oil may help people with IBS-D deal with their symptoms.

How Peppermint Can be Consumed

- ❖ Peppermint Oil Capsules: Enteric-coated peppermint oil capsules are a popular way to help with IBS symptoms. The enteric layer keeps heartburn and acid reflux from happening.
- ❖ Tea with Peppermint: Some people may feel better after drinking peppermint tea made from fresh or dried leaves.

Safety and Ideas to think about, peppermint is safe for most people to take in small amounts.

Potential Side Effects: Some people may get heartburn or irritation from peppermint oil pills, especially if they are not enteric-coated.

When someone is allergic, they might react badly to peppermint. Reactions due to allergies are possible, but not common.

Drug interactions: Peppermint oil may not work well with some medicines. Talk to a doctor or nurse if you are taking drugs.

• **Uses in cooking**: Peppermint is often used in savory meals, desserts, and teas.

Some people with IBS may feel better after smelling peppermint, but it's important to remember that everyone reacts differently. If you have severe or ongoing digestive problems, you should talk to a doctor or nurse to get a full review and the right advice. Without proper medical supervision, peppermint or peppermint oil should not be used instead of medicines that a doctor has recommended.

5. Garlic is good for your heart

Even though garlic might be good for your heart, it's best to eat it as part of a healthy diet instead of just taking pills. While making any changes to your food or way of life, it's best to talk to a doctor first, especially if you already have heart problems or are on medication. Without proper medical supervision, garlic supplements should not be used instead of medicines that your doctor has recommended.

For hundreds of years, people have known that garlic (Allium sativum) might be good for your heart. A lot of studies show that garlic might be good for a lot of different heart factors. Garlic may lower the risk of blood clots by taking action against platelets.

Compounds that work:

There is something called allicin that is made when garlic is crushed or chopped. It is thought to be a key bioactive molecule that might be good for the heart.

❖ **Sulfur Compounds**: Garlic has many sulfur-containing compounds, such as diallyl disulfide, diallyl trisulfide, and others. These compounds give garlic its smell and may have health benefits.

- ❖ **Vasodilation:** Allicin may help relax blood vessels, which means it has vasodilatory benefits. This might help bring down blood pressure.
- ❖ **Nitric Oxide Production**: Garlic may increase the production of nitric oxide, a chemical that makes blood vessels wider and better at moving blood through them.
- ❖ **Reduction in LDL Cholesterol**: Garlic may help lower amounts of low-density lipoprotein (LDL) cholesterol, the type of cholesterol that your body makes.

Garlic may have a small effect on cutting triglyceride levels.

- ❖ Anti-Inflammatory and Antioxidant Effects: Garlic has been studied for its possible anti-inflammatory effects, which can be good for heart health.
- ❖ Antioxidant Properties: Antioxidants found in garlic may help fight free radicals and lower oxidative stress.

Forms of Consumption

If you want to eat fresh garlic, you can usually add it to food, which tastes great.

Nutritional Supplements: For people who want a stronger form, there are nutritional supplements like garlic oil pills, aged garlic extract, and garlic powder capsules.

Studies show that garlic may slow the development of atherosclerosis, which is the hardening and narrowing of arteries. This can help prevent cardiovascular disease.

A lower chance of cardiovascular events has been linked to eating garlic in some groups, though the evidence is not always strong.

An average amount of garlic as part of a healthy diet is thought to be safe for most people.

Some medicines, especially those that thin the blood, may not work well with garlic pills. Especially if you are taking medications, you should talk to a medical worker.

6. Valerian

People have long used Valerian (Valeriana officinalis) because it may help with sleep problems and make you feel more relaxed. Read on to learn more about valerian and how it can help with sleep problems:

Valerian extract can help with insomnia and other sleep problems.

Compounds that do work:

- ❖ Valerenic acid is thought to be the main active ingredient in valerian and is linked to the calming benefits of the plant.
- ❖ Valerene is another chemical that can be found in valerian. It may also help with its calming benefits.
- ❖ Effects that help you sleep: calming and sedative: Valerian is thought to have mild sedative and anxiolytic (for anxiety) effects that may help people relax and get a better night's sleep.
- ❖ Gamma-aminobutyric acid (GABA) receptors in the brain may combine with valerenic acid. GABA receptors are linked to calming effects.

Valerian's possible effects on enhancing the quality of sleep and decreasing the amount of time needed to fall asleep have been the subject of research into its use in the treatment of insomnia and other sleep disorders.

Some people find that valerian helps them sleep better when they're having trouble falling or staying asleep.

• **Consumption Methods**: One popular way to take valerian root is to make tea from dried root. Its slightly bitter and earthy flavor has made this tea famous.

You can get valerian supplement in the form of capsules, pills, or tinctures.

Results of the Study: While valerian has shown promise in a number of trials for enhancing the quality of sleep, the findings have been inconsistent, and people react differently to the herb.

Valerian is most typically prescribed for short-term usage, and you may start to feel its benefits after just a few weeks of regular use.

• **Safety and Things to Think About**: when taken as directed, valerian has no health risks to the average person. Mild side effects, such as dizziness or stomach distress, are possible.

Potential Drug Interactions: Valerian has the potential to interact with sedatives and liver-affecting drugs, among others. Talk to your doctor, particularly if you are on any kind of medicine.

Culinary Uses:

> ❖ **Valerian in the Kitchen**: The powerful and somewhat unpleasant aroma of valerian makes it an uncommon ingredient in cooking.
> ❖ **Reaction:** valerian works differently for people. Sleep quality may improve dramatically for some people and significantly worse for others.

Please consult a medical expert before using valerian for any long-term sleep problems; it is not a replacement for their advise or treatment.

Talk to a doctor for an in-depth assessment and individualized advice if you can't seem to shake chronic sleep problems or suspect you have a medical concern. Never take a valerian supplement in place of a doctor-prescribed medicine without first consulting your doctor.

7. Lavender

The aromatic herb lavender (Lavandula spp.) has a long history of use, including as a stress reliever and a means of relaxation due to its pleasant aroma.

Anxiety, tension, and sleeplessness are some of the conditions that lavender can help with.

Gathering Materials: Sachets of lavender, essential oil for diffusion, or a cup of lavender tea.

Additional information regarding lavender and its possible impact on stress and anxiety is provided below:

Active compounds:

> ❖ Linalool is one of the key components of lavender oil and is thought to contribute to its relaxing and sedative properties.

❖ Linalyl acetate: Another chemical discovered in lavender, linalyl acetate, is linked to the floral scent and putative calming qualities.

Aromatherapy:

Lavender can promote relaxation and calmness. Inhaling the scent may provide rapid relaxing benefits.Some research suggest that lavender has modest sedative properties, which contribute to its ability to reduce anxiety and promote relaxation.

Clinical studies on reducing anxiety and stress, while research is ongoing, several studies suggest that lavender may help relieve anxiety and stress symptoms.

Stress Response: Lavender may affect the autonomic nerve system, potentially lowering the body's stress response.

Forms of Use:

Some common ways to use lavender essential oil are as an essential oil or in a blend with other oils. It can be circulated, mixed with bath water, or put on the skin after being diluted with a carrier oil.

❖ Lavender Tea: Another way to enjoy the possible calming benefits of lavender is to add dried flowers to tea.
❖ Lavender Supplements: You can also buy capsules that contain lavender oil.
❖ Aromatherapy for Sleep: One popular way to help people sleep is to diffuse lavender oil or use products that smell like lavender in their bedroom.

Overall, lavender is safe for most people as long as they follow the directions on how to use it. However, some people may be allergic to the smell or have skin irritations when they come into direct touch with lavender oil that hasn't been diluted.

Pregnancy: Women who are pregnant should be careful and talk to a doctor before using lavender items, especially concentrated ones.

Interactions: Some medicines may not work well with lavender remedies. Talk to a medical worker, especially if you are taking medicines.

Lavender can have different effects on different people. For example, while many people find it relaxing, it might not have the same effect on everyone.

• **In the kitchen:** Lavender is used in the kitchen, mostly for baking and cooking. It adds a unique floral taste to food.

Lavender can help you deal with stress and worry, but you should only use it in small amounts and be aware of how sensitive different people are. If your anxiety feelings don't go away or get worse, you should talk to a doctor or nurse to get a full diagnosis and the right treatment. Lavender products should not be used instead of prescription drugs without the right medical care.

8. St. John's Wort

Herbal medicine called St. John's Wort (Hypericum perforatum) has been used for hundreds of years to treat a wide range of illnesses, including mild to moderate sadness. It is a flowering plant with yellow petals that grows wild in many parts of the world, including Europe, Asia, and North America. It has a long history of medicinal use, particularly in traditional European herbalism.

The plant's active constituents include hypericin and hyperforin, among others. These compounds are believed to have antidepressant and anti-inflammatory properties. St. John's Wort has been used traditionally to treat a variety of ailments, including depression, anxiety, wounds, burns, and inflammation.

Ways to use St John's Wort

❖ **Capsules or Tablets:** St. John's Wort extract is often available in capsule or tablet form, standardized to contain a specific amount of the active ingredients, such as hypericin and hyperforin. This form allows for easy and precise dosing.

❖ **Tinctures:** Tinctures are concentrated liquid extracts made by soaking St. John's Wort in alcohol or another solvent. They are typically taken orally by diluting a few drops in water or juice. Tinctures can provide a potent and fast-acting way to consume St. John's Wort.

❖ **Tea:** Dried St. John's Wort flowers and leaves can be brewed into a tea. Simply steep a teaspoon of dried herb in hot water for about 10 minutes, then strain and drink. This method provides a soothing and gentle way to consume the herb, although it may not be as concentrated as other forms.

❖ **Topical Preparations:** St. John's Wort extract can be applied topically to the skin in the form of creams, ointments, or oils. This application is commonly used to help heal wounds, bruises, burns, and inflammatory skin conditions.
However, it's essential to avoid sun exposure after applying St. John's Wort topically, as it can increase sensitivity to sunlight and cause sunburn.

❖ **Infused Oil:** St. John's Wort extract can be infused into carrier oils, such as olive oil or almond oil, to create a topical oil that can be applied directly to the skin. This infused oil is particularly useful for massage or for treating minor skin irritations.

❖ **Powder:** St. John's Wort extract is sometimes available in powdered form, which can be mixed into smoothies, juices, or other beverages. However, the taste of the powder can be bitter, so it may be less palatable than other forms.

❖ **Short-Term Use**: Users are often told to only use St. John's Wort for a short time. Because of possible side effects and conflicts, long-term use may not be a good idea.

❖ **Generally Safe**: Many people think that St. John's Wort is safe to use as advised.

❖ **Side Effects**: Some side effects could be stomach problems, feeling dizzy, or being sensitive to sunshine.

❖ **Interactions**: Oral contraceptives, antidepressants, and blood thinners are some of the medicines that St. John's Wort can combine with. Certain medicines may not work as well if you take it.

❖ **Not Good for People with Severe Depression**: People with severe depression shouldn't take St. John's Wort. People who are having suicidal ideas or major depressive episodes should see a doctor.

❖ **Response of Each Individual:** Each person may react differently to St. John's Wort, and how well it works may rest on things like how depressed they are and their own biochemistry.

- ❖ **Meeting with a medical professional:** Speaking to a doctor or nurse before using St. John's Wort is very important, especially if you are on medicine or already have a health problem.

Without proper medical supervision, St. John's Wort should not be used instead of medicines that a doctor has recommended.

Some people with mild to severe depression may feel better after taking St. John's Wort, but it's important to be careful and talk to a doctor before starting to use it. Depression is a serious illness, and it's important to get a full evaluation from a doctor before choosing the right treatment.

9. Ginkgo biloba

Ginkgo biloba is one of the oldest living tree species, dating back over 200 million years. It's also one of the most widely studied and used herbal supplements in the world. The extract of ginkgo leaves is often taken orally and is believed to offer a range of health benefits.

Ginkgo biloba supplements are available in various forms, including capsules, tablets, liquid extracts, and teas. It's essential to follow the recommended dosage instructions and consult with a healthcare professional before starting any new supplement, especially if you have underlying health conditions or are taking medications, as ginkgo biloba may interact with certain drugs.

Additionally, pregnant or breastfeeding women should avoid ginkgo biloba supplements due to potential risks.

How ginkgo biloba can help

- ❖ **Memory and Cognitive Function**: Ginkgo biloba is perhaps best known for its potential to improve memory and cognitive function. Some studies suggest that it may help enhance mental alertness, concentration, and memory in both young and elderly individuals. It's often used as a natural remedy to support brain health and to help manage symptoms of age-related cognitive decline.

- ❖ **Peripheral Circulation**: Ginkgo biloba extract is thought to improve blood flow, particularly to the brain and extremities. This improved circulation may benefit individuals with conditions such as intermittent claudication (painful leg cramping due to poor circulation) and Raynaud's disease (a condition that causes reduced blood flow to the extremities).

- ❖ **Antioxidant Properties**: Ginkgo biloba contains antioxidants, including flavonoids and terpenoids, which help neutralize harmful free radicals in the body. These antioxidants may help protect cells from damage caused by oxidative stress and inflammation, potentially reducing the risk of chronic diseases.

- ❖ **Vision and Eye Health:** Some research suggests that ginkgo biloba may support vision and eye health by improving blood flow to the eyes and protecting against age-related macular degeneration (AMD) and glaucoma. However, more studies are needed to confirm these effects.

- ❖ **Anxiety and Depression:** Ginkgo biloba has been investigated for its potential to alleviate symptoms of anxiety and depression. While some studies have shown promising results, the evidence is not conclusive, and more research is needed in this area.

More research needs to be done on Ginkgo biloba to see if it can really help brain health and mind function. Some studies show possible benefits, especially when it comes to memory loss and slight cognitive decline. Other studies, on the other hand, show mixed or no results at all. You should be careful when taking Ginkgo biloba and think about your health and any possible reactions. This is true for any herbal product.

Talk to a healthcare professional for specialized help. Study after study is still telling us more about how Ginkgo biloba can help brain health. This is why people are still interested in and looking into it.

Dosage:

- ❖ **Standardized Extracts**: These are usually sold in standardized extracts that have set amounts of active ingredients.The daily dose can be anywhere from 120 mg to 240 mg.

Instructions for administration:

- ❖ **When to take it**: Ginkgo is often taken with food to help the body absorb it better.
- ❖ **Consistency**: It is often suggested that you use something consistently for a long time.

Effects on the body:

- ❖ **Gastrointestinal Distress**: Some people may have mild problems with their digestion.
- ❖ **Allergic responses**: Allergic responses have only happened a few times.
- ❖ **Blood Thinners**: Ginkgo may not work well with blood thinners.
- ❖ **Seizure Threshold**: People who have had seizures in the past should be careful.

10. Milk Thistle for Liver Health:

Milk thistle (Silybum marianum) is a flowering herbal remedy that has been used for centuries, particularly in traditional European medicine, for various health purposes. One of its primary applications is in promoting liver health.

Milk thistle has gained popularity as a natural remedy for liver health, and research continues to explore its potential benefits. While it's generally regarded as safe and well-tolerated, individual responses may vary. For those considering milk thistle supplementation, particularly for specific liver conditions, consultation with healthcare professionals is recommended. The evolving scientific understanding of milk thistle's mechanisms and efficacy underscores the importance of evidence-based approaches in leveraging herbal remedies for liver health.

Here's a detailed exploration of milk thistle for liver health:

Conditions: Liver disorders and detoxification.

Preparation: Milk thistle supplements.

Botanical Background:

❖ Plant Description: Milk thistle is characterized by its spiky purple flowers and distinctive white veins.

Active Compound:

❖ Silymarin is the key bioactive component, comprised of several flavonolignans.

Mechanisms of Action:

❖ Antioxidant Properties: Silymarin as an Antioxidant: Acts as a powerful antioxidant, neutralizing free radicals.

❖ Cellular Protection: Protects liver cells from oxidative stress and damage.

Anti-Inflammatory Effects:

❖ Modulating Inflammation: Silymarin has been shown to have anti-inflammatory effects.

❖ Reducing Inflammatory Markers: May decrease markers of inflammation in the liver.

Liver Conditions and Disorders:

❖ Liver Detoxification Support: Enhancing Detoxification Pathways: Milk thistle is believed to support the liver's natural detoxification processes.

❖ Protecting Hepatocytes: Silymarin may help protect liver cells from toxins.

❖ Fibrosis Reduction: Some studies suggest that milk thistle may help reduce liver fibrosis.

Non-Alcoholic Fatty Liver Disease (NAFLD):

Reducing Fat Accumulation:

•Hepatoprotective Effects: Silymarin may have protective effects against fatty liver disease.

•Insulin Sensitivity: Some research suggests improved insulin sensitivity.

Clinical Significance:

•Varied Outcomes: While some studies show improvements, others have more mixed results.

Liver Regeneration and Repair:

•Stimulating Regeneration:

•Cell Proliferation: Silymarin may stimulate the regeneration of liver cells.

•Potential for Healing: This property is particularly relevant after liver damage.

Post-Surgery Recovery:

•Supporting Healing Process: Milk thistle is sometimes used post-surgery or after liver-related interventions.

Consultation Recommended: Individual cases should be discussed with healthcare professionals.

Dosage and Administration:

•Silymarin Content: Dosages are often based on the percentage of silymarin in standardized extracts.

•Common dosages range from 140 mg to 420 mg per day.

Administration Guidelines:

•Timing and Consistency: It's often recommended to take milk thistle with meals for better absorption.

•Duration of Use: Extended use may be considered in certain cases, but consultation is advised.

11. Aloe Vera for Skin Conditions:

One common natural medicine is aloe vera, which can be used for a variety of skin ailments due to its adaptability and possible advantages. Aloe vera's natural chemicals are responsible for its medicinal properties, which can be utilized to alleviate sunburn, moisturize dry skin, or treat certain dermatological problems.

People with sensitive skin or allergies should proceed with caution, since individual reactions can differ. When dealing with severe or long-lasting skin issues, it is best to seek the advice of a dermatologist or other qualified healthcare provider for specific recommendations.

The succulent aloe vera plant has a rich history in traditional medicine due to its healing qualities. Its leaf gel has gained a lot of attention due to its possible usefulness in treating a wide range of skin disorders. If you want to know how to use aloe vera to keep your skin healthy, here it is:

Environmental Botany:

The most popular species of aloe vera for therapeutic uses is Aloe barbadensis Miller.

Vegetable plant known as a succulent has thick, fleshy leaves that contain a gel-like material.

Important Parts and Processes:

- ❖ **Leaf Structure:** Aloe vera leaves are composed of several layers, including the outer rind, the latex layer (found just beneath the outer rind), and the inner gel. The outer rind is tough and contains cells that help prevent water loss from the plant. The inner gel is the clear, mucilaginous substance found inside the leaf and is rich in nutrients and bioactive compounds.
- ❖ Biochemical Composition: Aloe vera gel contains a variety of bioactive compounds, including polysaccharides, vitamins, minerals, amino acids, enzymes, and antioxidants.The primary active components of aloe vera gel are polysaccharides, particularly acemannan, which has immune-stimulating properties and may contribute to the plant's therapeutic effects.

Processes within Aloe Vera

- ❖ **Photosynthesis**: Like other plants, aloe vera undergoes photosynthesis, a process by which it uses sunlight to convert carbon dioxide and water into glucose (sugar) and oxygen.

- ❖ **Synthesis of Bioactive Compounds:** Aloe vera synthesizes various bioactive compounds within its cells, including polysaccharides, antioxidants, and enzymes, which contribute to its medicinal properties.
- ❖ **Water Transport:** Aloe vera plants have specialized vascular tissues that transport water and nutrients throughout the plant, allowing them to thrive in arid conditions.
- ❖ **Healing and Defense Mechanisms:** When aloe vera leaves are damaged or wounded, the plant activates defense mechanisms to protect itself and promote healing. This may involve the synthesis and release of bioactive compounds that have antibacterial, anti-inflammatory, and wound-healing properties.

What Is in Aloe Vera Gel?

Acemannan is one example of a polysaccharide that has immune-modulating characteristics.

Amylase and lipase are two examples of enzymes that can improve digestion and skin condition.

• Antioxidants: Fighting oxidative stress and free radicals.

Mechanisms of Action:

- ❖ Anti-Inflammatory Effects: Aloe vera may help reduce inflammation in the skin.
- ❖ Wound Healing: Accelerating the healing process for minor wounds and burns.
- ❖ Moisturizing Properties: Hydrating and soothing dry or irritated skin.

Common Uses for Skin Conditions:

- ❖ Sunburn Relief
- ❖ Cooling Sensation: Aloe vera provides a cooling effect on sunburned skin.
- ❖ Reducing Inflammation: Helps alleviate redness and inflammation.

Minor Burns and Wounds:

- ❖ Wound Healing: Aloe vera may enhance the healing of minor cuts and burns.
- ❖ Reducing Scar Formation: Potential for minimizing scarring.

Skin Moisturization and Hydration:

- ❖ Dry Skin Conditions: Hydrating Properties: Aloe vera is a natural moisturizer for dry skin.
- ❖ Improving Skin Elasticity: Enhances the skin's flexibility and suppleness.
- ❖ Eczema and Psoriasis: Soothing Irritation: Aloe vera's anti-inflammatory properties can provide relief.
- ❖ Reducing Itchiness: May alleviate itching associated with these conditions.

Acne and Blemishes:

- ❖ Anti-Inflammatory: Helps reduce inflammation associated with acne.
- ❖ Antibacterial Properties: Aloe vera may have antibacterial effects.

Scar Reduction:

- ❖ Promoting Healing: Aloe vera gel may aid in minimizing acne-related scars.

Application Techniques: Regular and consistent use is typically recommended.

Dermatitis and Allergic Reactions:

- ❖ Soothing Effects:
- ❖ Calming Irritated Skin: Aloe vera may soothe dermatitis or allergic reactions.
- ❖ Antipruritic Properties: Relieves itching associated with skin allergies.

Skin Aging and Wrinkles:

- ❖ Collagen Stimulation: Some studies suggest aloe vera may stimulate collagen production.
- ❖ Reducing Wrinkles: Potential benefits in reducing fine lines and wrinkles.

Antioxidant Protection:

- ❖ Combatting Free Radicals: Aloe vera's antioxidants may protect against oxidative stress.
- ❖ UV Radiation: Potential for protecting the skin from sun damage.

Application and Safety:

- ❖ Gel Usage: Directly applying aloe vera gel to the skin.
- ❖ Creams and Lotions: Commercial products with aloe vera as a key ingredient.

Potential Allergic Reactions:

- ❖ Patch Testing: Important for individuals with sensitive skin or allergies.
- ❖ Rare Side Effects: Allergic reactions are uncommon but can occur.

Chapter 6

Herbal Support for Digestion

For a long time, people have turned to herbs as a means to aid digestion, alleviate gas, and fix other gastrointestinal problems.

It's best to check with a doctor or herbalist before taking any herb, especially if you have a history of gastrointestinal issues or are taking any kind of medicine, because everyone reacts differently to herbs. In addition to using these herbs, a varied and balanced diet can help with digestive health in general.

Herbs that aid digestion include the following:

1. **Peppermint**, scientifically known as Mentha piperita, has several health benefits, including the alleviation of indigestion, gas, and gastrointestinal spasms. Peppermint essential oil is available in two forms: tea and an inhalable or topical diluted form.
2. **Zingiber officinale**, or ginger, has anti-nausea, pro-digestive, and anti-inflammatory properties. Fresh ginger in a variety of forms, including drinks, pills, and seasonings for food.
3. **Chamomile**, or Matricaria chamomilla, is a herb that helps with indigestion, gas, and digestive calmness.Chamomile can be consumed in two forms: tea and supplements.
4. **Fennel:** Foeniculum vulgare contains carminative qualities, aids digestion, and reduces gas. Options: fennel seeds, fennel supplements, or fennel tea.
5. **Licorice Root (Glycyrrhiza glabra):**

   Benefits: Supports overall digestive function and may help with indigestion and heartburn.

   Forms: Licorice tea, deglycyrrhizinated licorice (DGL) supplements.

6. **Turmeric (Curcuma longa):**

Benefits: Anti-inflammatory properties can help with conditions like irritable bowel syndrome (IBS).

Forms: Turmeric supplements, turmeric-infused dishes.

7. Artichoke (Cynara scolymus):

Benefits: Stimulates bile production, aiding digestion and relieving indigestion.

Forms: Artichoke leaf extract supplements.

8. Gentian (Gentiana lutea):

Benefits: Stimulates digestive juices, supporting overall digestion.

Forms: Gentian root supplements.

9. Dandelion (Taraxacum officinale):

Benefits: Supports liver health and aids digestion by promoting bile production.

Forms: Dandelion tea, dandelion root supplements.

10. Meadowsweet (Filipendula ulmaria):

Benefits: Soothes and protects the digestive tract, reducing acidity.

Forms: Meadowsweet tea, meadowsweet supplements.

11. Aloe Vera (Aloe barbadensis miller):

Benefits: Supports digestive health, particularly for soothing and healing the gut lining.

Forms: Aloe vera juice (internally consumed, ensuring it's labelled for internal use).

12. Coriander (Coriandrum sativum):

Benefits: Relieves gas, bloating, and indigestion.

Forms: Coriander seeds in teas or as a spice in meals.

13. Cumin (Cuminum cyminum):

Benefits: Aids digestion, reduces bloating, and may alleviate symptoms of irritable bowel syndrome (IBS).

Forms: Cumin seeds in teas or as a spice in meals.

14. Cardamom (Elettaria cardamomum):

Benefits: Eases indigestion, supports overall digestive health.

Forms: Cardamom seeds in teas or as a spice in meals.

Herbal Support for Diabetes

You should still see a doctor if you're having trouble controlling your diabetes, although some herbs may help. Close collaboration between healthcare providers and people with diabetes is essential for the safe and effective management of the disease.

Keep in mind that herbs might have different effects on different people and that they can combine with other drugs. Before using herbs as part of a diabetic control plan, it is important to talk to your doctor. Important parts of diabetes care also include managing stress, eating healthily, and exercising regularly.

Research on the possible advantages of the following herbs for diabetes management has been conducted:

1. **Cinnamon:** One possible benefit of cinnamon (Cinnamomum verum) is that it may reduce blood sugar levels and increase insulin sensitivity.

Various forms include cinnamon supplements and cinnamon added to food.

2. **Benefits of Bitter Melon (Momordica charantia)** include the presence of chemicals that may reduce blood sugar levels.

You can find bitter melon in a variety of forms, including supplements, juice, and food.

3. **Fenugreek**, whose scientific name is Trigonella foenum-graecum, may have a positive effect on glucose metabolism and blood sugar regulation.

Consumption: fenugreek seeds, dietary supplements, or spiced food.

4. **Ginseng (Panax ginseng):** Advantages: Research indicates that ginseng may help improve insulin sensitivity.

Consumption: Ginseng tea or dietary supplements.

5. **Curcumin,** the active ingredient in turmeric (Curcuma longa), may have benefits that regulate blood sugar levels and reduce inflammation.

There are two main forms of turmeric: pills and food.

6. **Aloe Vera (Aloe barbadensis miller):**

Benefits: Some studies suggest potential blood sugar-lowering effects.

Forms: Aloe vera juice (internally consumed, ensuring it's labeled for internal use).

7. **Berberine (Berberis vulgaris):**

Benefits: May help lower blood sugar levels and improve insulin sensitivity.

Forms: Berberine supplements.

8. **Gymnema Sylvestre:**

Benefits: Known as the "sugar destroyer," it may help reduce sugar absorption in the intestines.

Forms: Gymnema supplements.

9. **Bilberry (Vaccinium myrtillus):**

Benefits: Contains anthocyanins that may have potential blood sugar-lowering effects.

Forms: Bilberry supplements or as a fruit.

10. **Holy Basil (Ocimum sanctum):**

Benefits: Some studies suggest potential benefits in reducing blood sugar levels.

Forms: Holy basil supplements or as a tea.

11. **Nettle (Urtica dioica):**

Possible benefits include increased insulin sensitivity and reduced blood sugar levels.

Supplements made from nettles or even as a tea.

12. **Cumin (Cuminum cyminum**): A few studies have shown that cumin may help improve insulin sensitivity.

You can use cumin seeds as a spice or in a tea.

13.**Garlic (Allium sativum):** Potentially beneficial for cardiovascular health and decreasing blood sugar levels.

Garlic comes in two forms: fresh garlic and supplements.

Herbal Support for Dementia

A lot of study is being done on herbal treatments for mental health problems like dementia. When using herbal treatments for dementia, you should be very careful. Also, you should know that there is no fix for the disease yet. If you are thinking about taking herbal remedies, you should always talk to a doctor first. This is very true when it comes to diseases like dementia.

People with dementia should be extra careful when thinking about taking plant medicines to help their minds. Since everyone reacts differently, these herbs shouldn't be thought of as an alternative to regular medical care. Because herbal medicines and medicines can sometimes mix badly with each other, you should always talk to a doctor before using any herbal medicines. Some important habits that can help keep your brain healthy are eating well, working out daily, and spending time with friends and family.

Some plants that have shown promise as brain boosters are:

1. Ginkgo Biloba may help your brain get more blood, which may help you think and remember things better.
2. Curcumin, the main chemical in turmeric (Curcuma longa), may be good for brain health because it fights inflammation and free radicals.Turnip comes in two main forms: pills and food.
3. Centella asiatica, which is another name for Gotu Kola. People have used it for a long time to improve brain health and cognitive function. Gotu kola comes in two different forms: tea and vitamins.
4. Bacopa Monnieri (Bacopa) is that it may help with memory and may even improve cognitive skills.

5. Sage, or Salvia officinalis, may improve memory and brain power because it has chemicals that do this.Sage comes in two forms: as a supplement and as a cooking plant.
6. Rosemary (Rosmarinus officinalis): Aromatic compounds may help your brain and make you more alert.Rosemary comes in many forms, such as essential oil, supplements, and vegetable that has been cooked.

A lot of study is being done on herbal treatments for mental health problems like dementia. When using herbal treatments for dementia, you should be very careful. Also, you should know that there is no fix for the disease yet. If you are thinking about taking herbal remedies, you should always talk to a doctor first. This is very true when it comes to diseases like dementia.

Herbal Remedy For High Blood Pressure

It's important to remember that even though some herbs may help lower blood pressure, you should always talk to a doctor before using any herbal treatments, especially if you already have a health problem or are on medication. Herbal treatments shouldn't be used instead of prescription drugs without first talking to a doctor or nurse.

Following are some herbs that have long been linked to possibly lowering blood pressure:

1. Hawthorn (Crataegus):

The plant hawthorn (Crataegus) has been used for hundreds of years in traditional medicine, mostly in Europe and Asia, to help keep the heart healthy. Most of the medical use of hawthorn is based on its possible benefits for heart diseases like high blood pressure. Hawthorn has been used for a long time to help keep the heart healthy, and some studies show it may also help lower blood pressure

 Here are some more facts about hawthorn:

•Some of the flavonoids found in hawthorn are rutin, quercetin, and hyperoside. These are thought to help the heart health.

•Proanthocyanidins are antioxidants that can be found in hawthorn may help protect blood vessels.

Effects on the heart and lungs

* Vasodilation: Hawthorn is thought to help make blood vessels bigger, which can help lower blood pressure. This might be because it can increase the production of nitric oxide, a chemical that makes blood vessels open.
* Heart performance: Hawthorn may be good for your heart's performance, including making heart contractions stronger, according to some studies.
* Keeping blood pressure in check: hawthorn can help lower blood pressure, but it's not all there, and more research is needed to be sure.

Duration of Use:

It's important to keep in mind that hawthorn may not show its effects on blood pressure right away. Long-term use may be better.

Types of Consumption:

One popular way to drink hawthorn tea is in a cup. Putting dried hawthorn leaves or berries in hot water will make tea.

- ❖ Extracts: You can also get liquid extracts and medicines, which are often used because they are easier to use.
- ❖ Capsules and tablets containing hawthorn extract can be purchased as dietary supplements.

Safety & Considerations:

Hawthorn is generally considered safe when used properly. However, it is critical to adhere to suggested quantities and check with a healthcare expert, particularly if you have pre-existing medical conditions or are taking drugs.

Potential Interactions: Hawthorn may interfere with certain drugs, especially those used to treat cardiac diseases. Always inform your healthcare practitioner if you are taking any herbal supplements.

Before using hawthorn or any other herbal therapy for high blood pressure, check with your doctor to confirm it is safe and appropriate for your individual health situation.

They can advise you on dose, any interactions, and evaluate your general cardiovascular health.

Examples of herbs to remedy high blood pressure

One food that may help lower blood pressure is garlic, scientifically known as Allium sativum. Relaxing blood arteries and increasing blood flow could be possible benefits.

Traditional medicine practitioners have long relied on the culinary and medicinal uses of the allium sativum plant, which includes garlic, to treat a wide range of ailments, including heart problems. In particular, allicin and other sulfur-containing chemicals in garlic are thought to have beneficial effects on cardiovascular health.

Additional information regarding garlic and its possible impact on blood pressure may be found here:

2. **Garlic (Allium sativum):** Research suggests garlic may reduce blood pressure. It may assist to relax blood arteries and increase blood flow.

Garlic (Allium sativum) is a common herb that has been used as both a culinary element and a traditional cure for a variety of health problems, including cardiovascular disease. Garlic's possible cardiovascular benefits are linked mostly to its active ingredient, allicin, and other sulfur-containing chemicals.

Here's additional information regarding garlic and its potential effects on blood pressure:

❖ Allicin and sulfur compounds:

Allicin is a chemical produced when garlic is crushed or diced. It has been investigated for its anti-inflammatory, antioxidant, and cardiovascular properties.

Sulfur Compounds: Garlic contains a variety of sulfur compounds, including diallyl disulfide, diallyl trisulfide, and others, which add to its distinctive odor and may provide health advantages.

• Allicin may relax blood arteries, resulting to decrease blood pressure.

Antioxidant Effects: Garlic's antioxidant qualities may help to improve cardiovascular health by lowering oxidative stress.

Clinical studies show mixed evidence. The evidence on garlic's usefulness in decreasing blood pressure is equivocal, and further research is needed to draw a firm conclusion.

3. **Olive leaf** refers to the leaves of the olive tree (Olea europaea), the same tree that produces olives and olive oil. Olive leaves have been used for centuries in traditional medicine for their potential health benefits.

Here's some information about olive leaf and its uses:

Olive leaf extract may help lower total and LDL cholesterol levels, according to some studies.

Effects on Inflammation: Olive leaf extract has been looked at to see if it has any effects on inflammation, which could be good for your heart health generally.

Antimicrobial Properties: • Antibacterial and Antiviral: Olive leaf extract has been shown to be antibacterial and antiviral, which may be why it was used in traditional medicine to boost the immune system.

How to Eat It: One way to eat olive leaf is to make tea from dried olive leaves. With this method, you can use the chemicals that dissolve in water to your advantage.

❖ Olive Leaf Extract: As a supplement, you can buy liquid extracts and pills that contain concentrated olive leaf extract.

Concerns and Safety: • Generally Safe: When used correctly, olive leaf extract is generally thought to be safe for most people. But different people may have different responses.

• **Possible Interactions**: Olive leaf extract might not work well with some medicines, like blood pressure medicines. Talk to a doctor or nurse, especially if you are on certain medicines or have certain health problems.

There are some problems with the research. Some studies show that olive leaf extract might be good for your heart, but more research is needed to be sure.

More research needs to be done on the best dose and long-term benefits of olive leaf extract.

It is very important to talk to a doctor before adding olive leaf extract or any other plant remedy to your routine, especially if you are trying to control your blood pressure. They can give you personalized information based on your health, the medicines you're taking, and any possible drug interactions. Without proper medical advice, herbal products should not be used instead of prescription drugs.

4. **Cinnamon (Cinnamomum)**: Cinnamon may have a small effect on blood pressure, according to certain studies. To prove its effectiveness, nevertheless, additional research is required.

For generations, people have relied on cinnamon for its flavor and, maybe, its medicinal powers. Although it shouldn't be used as a substitute for medical treatment, cinnamon has shown promise in a number of studies, particularly those pertaining to cardiovascular health and blood pressure. Cinnamon is further explained here:

Medicinal Substances:

The flavor and aroma of cinnamon are primarily caused by the major active component, cinnamonaldehyde. Potentially anti-inflammatory and antioxidant capabilities may also be present.

Some of cinnamon's purported health advantages may be due to its constituents, including cinnamonate and cinnamic acid.

- ❖ The Control of Blood Pressure:Cinnamon may help relax blood arteries and enhance blood flow by acting as a vasodilator.
- ❖ Cinnamon's antioxidant properties may help lower oxidative stress, which has been associated to heart problems.
- ❖ Enhancing Insulin Sensitivity and Its Relation to Blood Sugar: Cinnamon may have both direct and indirect positive effects on cardiovascular health, according to some research, by increasing insulin sensitivity and decreasing blood sugar levels.

Cinnamon Varieties:

Certified "true cinnamon" comes from the Cinnamomum verum tree and is known as Ceylon cinnamon. Many people suggest it for frequent usage because of its softer flavor.

The most common kind of cinnamon you'll find in most supermarkets is cassia cinnamon. It tastes harsher and has more coumarin, which, in excessive doses, could be harmful to the liver.

Consumption Methods:

• Ground Cinnamon: One simple and common approach to add cinnamon to your diet is to grind some cinnamon and add it to meals, drinks, or smoothies.

Spice up your cuisine with cinnamon sticks or steep them in boiling water for a refreshing cinnamon tea.

If you'd like a more potent cinnamon supplement, you can get it in the form of capsules or extracts. Dosage recommendations must be strictly adhered to.

Safety and Things to Think About:

• Mostly Safe: Most people think that cinnamon is safe when used as a spice in normal amounts. But taking too much cassia cinnamon, especially in supplement form, could expose you to coumarin and cause side effects.

• Possible Interactions: Cinnamon supplements might not work well with some medicines or make your blood thinner. Talk to a doctor or nurse, especially if you are on certain medicines or have certain health problems.

It is important to talk to a doctor before adding cinnamon or cinnamon tablets to your routine, especially if you are trying to control your blood pressure or other health issues. Based on your health, medicines, and possible drug interactions, they can give you advice. Cinnamon shouldn't be used instead of prescription drugs without the right medical guidance.

5. **Basil (Ocimum basilicum):** Compounds in basil may aid in blood vessel relaxation, which may help reduce blood pressure.

The fragrant herb basil (Ocimum basilicum) is a member of the mint family (Lamiaceae). Although it is commonly used in cooking, traditional medicine has long employed it for a number of health benefits. Although basil doesn't usually have a direct effect on blood pressure, it does contain substances that could improve cardiovascular health in general.

Here are some further details regarding basil:

• Active Compounds:

• Essential Oils: Eugenol, linalool, and citronellol are among the essential oils found in basil, which give it a unique scent and may offer health advantages.

• Flavonoids: Orientin and vicenin, two flavonoids with antioxidant qualities, are found in basil.

Effects of Antioxidants and Anti-Inflammators:

• Oxidative Stress: Basil contains antioxidants that may help counteract oxidative stress, which has been connected to a number of health problems, including heart disease.

• Anti-Inflammatory Properties: The anti-inflammatory properties of several chemicals found in basil, notably eugenol, have been researched.

Heart Health:

❖ Blood Vessel Relaxation: According to certain research, basil extracts may assist to relax blood vessels by having a vasodilatory action. This may help to keep blood pressure levels within a reasonable range.

❖ •Cholesterol Levels: Although there hasn't been much research done, there is some indication that basil may improve lipid profiles by lowering triglyceride and total cholesterol levels.

Types of consumption:

If you want to enjoy the taste and possible health benefits of fresh basil, you can add its leaves to salads, sandwiches, pasta, and other foods.

To make basil tea, you can put fresh or dried basil leaves in hot water and let them soak for a while. This might be a better way to get more of the phytochemicals that are good for you.

There are also basil supplements that come in capsules or extracts, though they are not very popular.

Generally Safe:

Most people can eat basil without getting sick as long as they don't eat too much of it and keep their diet balanced.

Basil may cause allergic reactions in some people, so it's important to be aware of any bad effects.

There aren't many interactions that basil can cause, but if you are pregnant, nursing, or taking medicine, you should talk to a doctor before using it.

Basil is an important part of many regional and international meals, such as Thai, Italian, and Mediterranean ones.

Soups, salads, sauces, and different meat and veggie dishes taste better with it.

It is important to remember that basil is not a replacement for prescription drugs for conditions like high blood pressure, even though it can be part of a healthy diet and may help with general health. Because everyone's health is different, it's best to talk to a doctor before using basil or any other herb as a remedy if you have specific health issues or are thinking about trying it.

6. Celery Seed (Apium graveolens):

Celery seed extract has been investigated for its potential antihypertensive effects. It may help lower blood pressure by improving blood vessel dilation.

Celery seed, derived from the Apium graveolens plant, is known for its distinct flavor and aroma and has been used traditionally for various medicinal purposes. While celery seed is often promoted for its potential health benefits, including blood pressure regulation, it's important to note that scientific evidence is limited, and more research is needed.

Here are more details about celery seed and its potential effects:

Active Compounds:

- ❖ Phthalides: Celery seeds contain phthalides, such as 3-n-butylphthalide (3nB), which are believed to contribute to its potential health effects.
- ❖ Apigenin: This is a flavonoid found in celery that has antioxidant properties.

Blood Pressure Control:

- ❖ Diuretic Effects: Studies on animals show that celery seed may have diuretic effects, which means it may make you pee more. By lowering the amount of fluid in the body, this might help lower blood pressure.
- ❖ Vasodilation: It has been claimed that celery seed may make blood vessels wider, which would help relax them and make blood flow better.

Forms of Consumption:

Whole celery seeds can be used in cooking, pickling, or as a spice to add flavor to dishes.

Celery Seed Extract: Extracts and supplements are available, providing a more concentrated form of celery seed.

Safety and Considerations:

Celery seed is considered safe for most people when consumed in moderation. However, individuals with celery allergies may experience adverse reactions.

Interactions:

Celery seed supplements may interact with certain medications, including those with blood-thinning effects. Consult with a healthcare professional, especially if you are taking medications or have specific health conditions.

Herbal Remedies for Common Ailments

Do keep in mind that herbal treatments may help some people, but you should talk to a doctor or nurse before using them, especially if you already have a health problem or are taking medicine. Herbal medicines can also have different effects on different people.These herbs can help with some common health problems

1. **The peppermint** plant (Mentha piperita) is often used to treat digestive problems like upset stomach, gas, and nausea.

Additional Information:

   - ❖ Peppermint tea, peppermint oil pills, or putting diluted peppermint oil on your skin are all good ways to use it.
   - ❖ Benefits: Peppermint can help relax the muscles in your digestive system, which can make gas and indigestion less painful.

2. **Camomile (Matricaria chamomilla):** Problems with digestion, insomnia, and stress are common.

Additional Information:

   - ❖ Use: Chamomile tea or pills that contain chamomile.
   - ❖ Benefits: Chamomile can help relax the digestive system and reduce inflammation. It's also known to help with worry and sleeplessness because it calms people down.

3. **Ginger, or Zingiber officinale** is often used to treat feeling sick, motion sickness, or inflammation are common symptoms.

More information:

   - ❖ Fresh ginger, ginger tea, or ginger pills.
   - ❖ Benefits: Ginger can help with motion sickness and makes you feel less sick. It may also help reduce inflammation because it has anti-inflammatory properties.

4. **Curcuma longa**, or turmeric: is often used to treat pain and swelling in the joints

More information:

   - ❖ Turmeric pills or cooking with turmeric are two ways to use it.

❖ Benefits: Curcumin, which is found in turmeric, is known to reduce inflammation. It might help ease joint pain and reduce swelling.

5. **Echinacea (Echinacea purpurea):** Flu, Cold, and Immune System Support. Use echinacea tea or take echinacea pills as directed.
   - ❖ Echinacea may help shorten the length and lessen the intensity of flu and cold symptoms by boosting the immune system.

6. **Valeriana officinalis:** Disorders of Sleep and Anxiety:
   - ❖ Dosage and Administration: Valerian root pills or tea.Some people find that valerian helps them sleep better and feel less anxious because of its modest sedative effects.

7. **Lavender, or Lavender oleifera**
   - ❖ Typical Symptoms: Restlessness, Worry, and Lack of Sleep
   - ❖ For aromatherapy purposes, try using lavender essential oil or brewing some lavender tea.
   - ❖ Lavender is commonly used to alleviate stress, anxiety, and induce relaxation because to its relaxing characteristics.

8. **Hypericum perforatum**, also known as St. John's Wort
   - ❖ Advantages: St. John's Wort may help with mild to moderate depression and is thought to have mood-enhancing qualities.

9. **Allium sativum, garlic**
   - ❖ Usage Instructions: • Raw garlic or garlic supplements for common ailments include cardiovascular health and immune system support.
   - ❖ Health Benefits: Garlic may help maintain heart health by reducing cholesterol levels and acting as an antibacterial.

10. **Cinnamon (Cinnamomum verum):** Managing Blood Sugar and Digestive Problems
    - ❖ Use cinnamon in cooking or take cinnamon pills for maximum effect.
    - ❖ The digestive system and blood sugar levels can both benefit from cinnamon's use.

These herbal medicines have gained a lot of recognition, but it's important to use them with caution and be mindful of any drug interactions or negative effects, particularly if you have a specific medical condition. If you are expecting a child, nursing a child, or have any other health concerns, you should talk to your doctor before using any herbal medicines

Chapter 7

Herbs for Stress Management

Researchers have found that some herbs may help relieve stress. It's important to remember that these herbs may help some people deal with worry, but everyone reacts differently. If you're thinking about using herbs to deal with stress, you should talk to a doctor first, especially if you already have a health problem or were prescribed medicine.

Here are some herbs that are often used to deal with stress:

1. **Ashwagandha, also known as Withania somnifera**: The best ways to use ashwagandha are in the form of vitamins, powdered root, or tea. This herb is an adaptogen, which means it may help the body deal with stress. The nervous system is thought to feel calmer after taking it.

2. **Rhodiola (Rhodiola rosea):** Rhodiola pills or tea are the best ways to use this herb.

   Benefits: This adaptogenic plant is known for its ability to make people less tired and better able to handle stress.

3. **Holy Basil (Ocimum sanctum)**: • Use holy basil tea, holy basil vitamins, or fresh holy basil leaves.

   Benefits: This herb is an adaptogen that may help with stress and nervousness. In ancient Ayurvedic medicine, it is also called Tulsi.

4. **Chamomile (Matricaria chamomilla)**:
   - ❖ Use: chamomile tea or chamomile pills.
   - ❖ Chamomile can help with stress and worry because it has mild calming effects and can help you relax.

5. **Lemon balm (Melissa officinalis).** You can use fresh lemon balm leaves, lemon balm tea, or lemon balm vitamins.
   - ❖ Benefits: This herb can help calm you down and may also have anxiety-lowering benefits. Mood may get better and worry may go down.

6. **Passionflower (Passiflora incarnata)**:
   - ❖ How to Use: herbs or tea made from passionflower.
   - ❖ Benefits: This plant is soothing and may help lower stress and increase relaxation.
7. Lavandula angustifolia, or lavender, is a plant that can be used in massage and to make lavender tea.
   - ❖ Lavender oil may help lower stress and anxiety when used in aromatherapy. Lavender tea can also help you relax.
8. **Valerian (Valeriana officinalis):** • Valerian root pills or valerian tea are good ways to use this plant.
   - ❖ Benefits: Valerian has mild calming benefits that may help you sleep and relax, which can help lower your stress.
9. **Ginseng (Panax ginseng):** • Take ginseng pills or drink ginseng tea.
   - ❖ Advantages: It is an adaptogenic herb that may help the body deal with stress better and improve general health.
10. **Use kava supplements or kava tea** (with caution owing to possible liver toxicity) as directed by a kava kava (Piper methysticum) expert.
    - ❖ **Advantage**s: for centuries, people in the South Pacific have relied on it to help them relax and cope with anxiety. Use it with caution and only under the supervision of a medical expert.
11. **Turmeric:**
    - ❖ How to Use: Supplements containing turmeric or using turmeric in cooking are two ways to use turmeric.
    - ❖ Benefits: It has curcumin, which may improve mood and reduce inflammation.
12. **Camellia sinensis, or green tea:**
    - ❖ Dosage and Administration: Hot or cold, straight or in supplement form.
    - ❖ Benefits: It has the amino acid L-theanine, which may help you relax and feel better overall.
13. **Rosemary (Rosmarinus officinalis):**
    - ❖ Application: Aromatherapy with rosemary essential oil or dietary supplements.
    - ❖ Possible stress reduction benefits of aromatherapy with rosemary oil.

14. Supplements containing **Hypericum perforatum**, also known as St. John's Wort, should be taken as directed.

   ❖ Advantages: It has a history of usage as a mood enhancer and shows promise in treating mild to moderate depression.

15. Ginkgo biloba (Ginkgo biloba) supplements

   ❖ Advantages: Ginkgo biloba is most famous for its positive effects on cognition, but it may also contain antioxidant qualities that improve health in general.

Make sure you select standardized herbal supplements of high quality and always take the dosages recommended. Herbal supplements might combine with other drugs or be harmful to people with certain health issues, so it's important to tell your doctor about them if you're taking any.

A well-rounded strategy for managing stress should include herbal medicines in addition to a healthy diet, frequent physical activity, and techniques for reducing stress like mindfulness or meditation.

Chapter 8

Herbal First Aid and Home Remedies

Herbal first aid and home remedies involve using natural ingredients, such as herbs, spices, and other plant-based substances, to address common health issues and minor injuries. While these remedies may not replace professional medical care for serious conditions, they can be effective for managing mild ailments and promoting overall wellness.

Here are some herbal first aid and home remedies for various health concerns:

1. **Wound Healing:**
   - ❖ Calendula: Calendula officinalis has antibacterial and anti-inflammatory properties. Infuse dried calendula flowers in oil to make a soothing salve or apply calendula cream to promote wound healing.
   - ❖ Aloe Vera: Aloe vera gel can be applied topically to minor cuts, burns, and abrasions to soothe irritation and promote healing.
   - ❖ Honey: Raw honey has antimicrobial properties and can be applied to wounds to prevent infection and accelerate healing.

2. **Digestive Issues:**
   - ❖ Peppermint: Peppermint (Mentha piperita) tea can help relieve symptoms of indigestion, bloating, and gas.
   - ❖ Ginger: Ginger (Zingiber officinale) tea or ginger capsules can help alleviate nausea, motion sickness, and digestive discomfort.
   - ❖ Chamomile: Chamomile (Matricaria chamomilla) tea has anti-inflammatory and calming properties that can help soothe an upset stomach and relieve digestive discomfort.

3. **Respiratory Conditions:**
   - ❖ Eucalyptus: Inhaling steam infused with eucalyptus essential oil can help relieve congestion and ease symptoms of respiratory infections such as colds and sinusitis.

❖ Thyme: Thyme (Thymus vulgaris) tea or thyme-infused honey can help soothe coughs and support respiratory health.

4. **Skin Irritations:**
   ❖ Lavender: Lavender (Lavandula angustifolia) essential oil has soothing properties that can help relieve itching, inflammation, and minor skin irritations. Dilute lavender oil with a carrier oil and apply it to affected areas.
   ❖ Oatmeal: Colloidal oatmeal can be added to bathwater to soothe itching and irritation associated with eczema, rashes, and insect bites.

5. **Pain Relief:**
   ❖ Arnica: Arnica (Arnica montana) gel or cream can be applied topically to relieve muscle aches, bruises, and inflammation.
   ❖ Willow Bark: Willow bark contains salicin, a compound similar to aspirin, which has pain-relieving and anti-inflammatory properties. Willow bark tea or supplements may help alleviate pain associated with headaches, muscle aches, and arthritis.

6. **Anxiety and Stress:**
   ❖ Lemon Balm: Lemon balm (Melissa officinalis) tea can help promote relaxation and reduce symptoms of anxiety and stress.
   ❖ Valerian: Valerian (Valeriana officinalis) root tea or supplements may help calm the nerves and promote better sleep.

When using herbal remedies, it's essential to research each herb's properties and potential interactions, as well as consult with a healthcare professional, especially if you have underlying health conditions, are pregnant or breastfeeding, or are taking medications. Additionally, always use caution and discontinue use if you experience any adverse reactions.

Chapter 9

Herbal Support for Women's Health

Herbs have been traditionally used to support various aspects of women's health, addressing issues such as hormonal balance, reproductive health, and overall well-being. It's important to note that while herbal remedies can be beneficial for some individuals, it's crucial to consult with a healthcare professional, especially for women with specific health concerns or conditions.

Here are some herbs commonly used for supporting women's health:

1. **Red Clover (Trifolium pratense):**

Benefits:

- ❖ Contains phytoestrogens, which may help balance estrogen levels.
- ❖ Traditionally used for menopausal symptoms and menstrual irregularities.

2. **Black Cohosh (Actaea racemosa):**

Benefits:

- ❖ Often used for managing menopausal symptoms, including hot flashes and mood swings.
- ❖ May have estrogen-like effects.

3. **Dong Quai (Angelica sinensis):**

Benefits:

- ❖ Commonly used in traditional Chinese medicine for menstrual issues and menopausal symptoms.
- ❖ Thought to support hormonal balance.

4. **Chaste Tree Berry (Vitex agnus-castus):**

Benefits:

- ❖ Supports hormonal balance, particularly in relation to the menstrual cycle.
- ❖ Used for conditions such as premenstrual syndrome (PMS) and irregular periods.

5. Ginger (Zingiber officinale):

Benefits:

- ❖ Anti-inflammatory properties may help with menstrual pain.
- ❖ Can be consumed as ginger tea or added to meals.

6. Licorice Root (Glycyrrhiza glabra):

Benefits:

- ❖ May support adrenal health and hormonal balance.
- ❖ Used in herbal blends for women's reproductive health.

7. Maca (Lepidium meyenii):

Benefits:

- ❖ Traditionally used for energy, stamina, and hormonal balance.
- ❖ May support reproductive health and libido.

8. Motherwort (Leonurus cardiaca):

Benefits:

- ❖ Often used for menstrual issues and to ease anxiety.
- ❖ May have calming effects on the nervous system.

9. Saw Palmetto (Serenoa repens):

Benefits:

- ❖ Primarily known for supporting prostate health, but also used for hormonal balance in women.
- ❖ May be helpful for conditions like polycystic ovary syndrome (PCOS).

10. Dandelion Root (Taraxacum officinale):

Benefits:

- ❖ Supports liver health, aiding in hormonal metabolism.
- ❖ May be used for conditions related to hormonal imbalances.

Note:

- ❖ Follow suggested dosages for herbal medicines and be mindful of any conflicts with pharmaceuticals or side effects. Before using herbs, see a healthcare practitioner, especially if you are pregnant, nursing, or have any specific health conditions.
- ❖ For best results, use high-quality, organic herbs.
- ❖ Individual Responses: Herbs can have varying effects and may take longer to show results.
- ❖ A holistic approach to women's health include a balanced diet, frequent exercise, and stress management, in addition to herbal medicines.

If you have specific health problems, always seek expert medical advice, and let your doctor know about any herbal supplements you are taking.

Fertility and Pregnancy

Herbs have long been used to aid with conception and pregnancy, but it is critical to utilize these cures with carefully and under the supervision of a healthcare practitioner. Before utilizing any herbs during fertility or pregnancy, consult a healthcare expert to determine their safety and suitability for your specific health problems.

The following herbs have been traditionally related with fertility and pregnancy support:

1. **Red Clover (Trifolium Pratense):**
   - ❖ High in phytoestrogens, which can improve hormonal balance. • \tTraditionally used to boost conception.
2. **Maca (Lepidium meyenii)** has adaptogenic characteristics and can improve hormonal balance. It has also been traditionally used to boost fertility and libido.
3. **Chaste Tree Berry (Vitex agnus-castus):** Promotes hormonal balance and controls the menstrual cycle. • Traditionally used for female reproductive health issues.
4. **Ginseng (Panax ginseng)** has adaptogenic properties and can improve reproductive health. It is also known to boost energy and vitality.
5. **Dong Quai** (Angelica sinensis) is used in traditional Chinese medicine to promote female reproductive health and support hormonal balance.

Herbs For Pregnancy Support

1. **Raspberry Leaf (Rubus idaeus)** is known for its uterine toning characteristics.Used during the second and third trimesters to support the uterus. May assist abbreviate labor.
2. **Nettle (Urtica dioica):** • High in vitamins and minerals, including iron. Improves overall nutrition during pregnancy.
3. **Ginger (Zingiber officinale):** Relieves nausea and morning sickness during pregnancy.Use in moderation.
4. **Peppermint (Mentha piperita):** • Can alleviate stomach discomfort during pregnancy. • Typically ingested as tea or in modest amounts.
5. **Chamomile (Matricaria chamomilla):** Calming and stress-relieving during pregnancy. Can be consumed as tea, but moderation is recommended.
6. **Lemon Balm (Melissa officinalis)** has relaxing effects and is used to alleviate tension and anxiety during pregnancy.
7. **Oatstraw (Avena sativa)** is a nutrient-rich herb that has traditionally been used to strengthen the neurological system during pregnancy. It can also be used as a herbal infusion.

Important Things to Keep in Mind:

❖ Talk to Your Doctor: Since everyone's fertility and pregnancy journey is unique, it's best to get a doctor's opinion before utilizing any herbs.

❖ Even herbs that are generally safe to use during pregnancy should still be used in moderation. Some plants might be harmful if taken in large quantities.

❖ Herb Quality: To Reduce Exposure to Pesticides and Other Contaminants, Use Herbs of High Quality That Are Organically Sourced.

When it comes to fertility and conception, a holistic approach includes more than just herbal therapies. Important parts include getting enough exercise, eating right, and getting prenatal care.

It's important to prioritize safety when taking herbs during pregnancy. Some herbs can cause unwanted side effects or combine with other medications. It is better to be safe than sorry.

In order to make sure that herbal supplements are used safely and appropriately, it is crucial for pregnant women or those attempting to conceive to collaborate closely with healthcare professionals, such as obstetricians, midwives, or fertility experts. For the sake of the mother's and the developing baby's health, expert advice is essential during every pregnancy.

Chapter 10

Build a First Aid Kit Containing Herbs

Compile remedies for common ailments such as minor burns, scrapes, and insect bites into a compact herbal first aid kit. Examples of herbal products used for first aid include calendula salve, lavender oil, and aloe vera gel.

❖ **Aromatherapy practice:**

Aromatherapy may employ herb-derived essential oils to promote relaxation, concentration, or upliftment of mood. To apply topically, dilute or diffuse essential oils within one's residence. Eucalyptus, lavender, and peppermint are all well-liked options.

❖ **Develop a routine**:

Incorporate the use of herbs into routine observances. Implementing rituals can help you incorporate herbal medicine into your daily life, whether it be by sipping herbal tea in the morning, applying herbal salve before bed, or integrating botanical scents into your yoga or meditation practice.

❖ **Developing One's Own Herbs**:

Small-scale herb cultivation at home is a viable option. One may be more inclined to integrate fresh herbs into their daily regimen of remedies and meals if they are easily accessible.

❖ **Observe Your Body Towards**:

Consider the effects that herbal remedies have on your body. It is critical to adapt one's herbal practices in accordance with the individual's condition, as each person is distinct.

Bear in mind that herbal medicine constitutes a supplementary methodology; therefore, it is imperative to seek guidance from a healthcare practitioner, particularly when dealing with particular health issues or while on medications. A deeper connection with nature can be fostered, and one's overall health and well-being can be bolstered through the gradual and pleasurable incorporation of herbal remedies into their daily routine.

Integrating herbal medicine into daily life involves incorporating natural remedies and practices to support overall health and well-being.

Here are practical ways to make herbal medicine a seamless part of your daily routine:

1.   **Morning Rituals:**

Herbal Tea: Have a cup of herbal tea to start your day. Herbs like ginger, chamomile, or peppermint can help with digestion and give you a little energy boost.

2.   **Kitchen Apothecary**:

Cooking with Herbs: Use culinary herbs like oregano, thyme, and rosemary to enhance the flavor and health benefits of your food.

Herbal Infusions: Herbs like turmeric and garlic can be used in cooking because they lower inflammation and boost the immune system.

3.   **Herb-Infused Water:**

Hydration Boost: For flavor and possible health benefits, add herbs like mint, cucumber, or citrus to your water.

4.   **Herbal Self-Care Products:**

Herbal Skincare: Use natural skincare products with calming and restorative qualities, such as calendula, lavender, or chamomile.

5.   Midday Herbal Break:

Snacks with herbal components: indulge in herbal-infused nuts or herbal energy balls, for example.

Tea Breaks: To unwind and revitalize yourself, take quick breaks throughout the day to sip herbal tea.

6.   **Herbal Supplements**:

Daily Tonics: You may want to include immune-stimulating or adaptogen-containing herbal supplements in your daily regimen.

7.   **Bedtime Rituals**:

Herbal Nightcap: Before going to bed, unwind with a soothing herbal tea like passionflower, valerian, or chamomile.

Herbal Pillow: To encourage sound sleep, stuff a sachet or pillow with dried herbs like chamomile or lavender.

8.   **Gardening with Medicinal Plants:**

Window Sill Garden: For easy access, grow a little herb garden with herbs like sage, basil, and mint on your window sill.

Outside Garden: If your garden has the room, include therapeutic herbs like lemon balm, calendula, and echinacea.

9.   **Herbal First Aid Kit:**

Make Your Own Salve: Assist minor wounds, bruises, and skin irritations with salves made from herbs such as calendula, comfrey, or arnica in a herbal first aid kit.

10.   **Mindful herbal practices**:

Herbal Meditation: To promote relaxation, add aromas of herbs, such as lavender or rosemary, to your meditation area.

Herbal Baths: For a calming and restorative experience, take an herbal bath using dried herbs or bath blends.

11.   **Educational Pursuits**:

Herbal Literature: To expand your knowledge, spend some leisure time reading books or articles about herbalism.

Online Courses: To deepen your knowledge of herbal medicine, look into online courses or attend workshops.

12.   **Herbal Community Engagement**:

Community Gardens: Take part in or lend support to community gardens that cultivate therapeutic herbs.

Herbal Workshops: To meet other herbal enthusiasts, go to local herbal workshops or sign up for internet forums.

13.   **Seasonal herbal practices**:

Seasonal Teas: Rotate herbal teas based on the seasons, incorporating herbs that align with the current weather or health needs.

14.   **Herbal Journaling**:

Reflection: Write in a journal about your experiences using various herbs, noting their effects and your general health.

15.   **Mindful Foraging**:

Wildcrafting: Get familiar with the wild herbs found in your area and include ethically harvested herbs in your daily regimen.

Keep in mind that incorporating herbal medicine into daily life requires consistency. You can find what works best for you and develop a sustainable, enjoyable herbal routine by introducing these practices gradually. Always seek the advice of a licensed herbalist or medical professional for specific guidance.

Chapter 11

Fundamental tenets of nutrient-dense, whole foods

These foods undergo minimal refining and processing in order to preserve as much of their natural state as feasible.

They are abundant in nutrients, encompassing a wide range of vital nutrients that are necessary for maintaining optimal health.

- **Balanced Macronutrients**: Whole foods that are high in nutrients usually have the right amount of carbs, proteins, and good fats.
  Adding a range of whole, nutrient-dense foods to a healthy, well-balanced diet can help you stay energetic, improve your health, and lower your risk of developing chronic diseases.

- **Anti-Inflammatory Foods**: The goal is to lower systemic inflammation, which is associated with a wide range of chronic diseases.
  Flaky fish (salmon, mackerel), ginger, turmeric, and leafy greens are a few examples. Consuming foods that contain anti-inflammatory properties can help alleviate inflammation in the body. Numerous medical issues, such as cardiovascular disease, diabetes, and autoimmune illnesses, are associated with chronic inflammation. If you want to improve your health and wellness in general, try eating more anti-inflammatory foods.
  Some important foods that reduce inflammation are detailed here:

- **Food Fish Rich in Fat:** Sardines, Mackerel, and Salmon: The anti-inflammatory effects of these fish are amplified by their high omega-3 fatty acid content. Omega-3s aid in cellular-level inflammation reduction.
- **Fruits**: berries: Anti-inflammatory blueberries, strawberries, and raspberries are rich in flavonoids, an antioxidant compound. Plus, they're a good source of vitamins and fiber.

- **Verdant Sprouts**: Among the many nutrients found in leafy greens like spinach, kale, and Swiss chard are antioxidants such as quercetin, a compound with anti-inflammatory effects.

- **Nuts:** The following nuts and seeds are rich in healthful fats, fiber, antioxidants, and flaxseed, chia, and almonds; the latter three also include alpha-linolenic acid (ALA), an anti-inflammatory compound.

- **Turmeric powder:** One of turmeric's key ingredients is curcumin, a powerful anti-inflammatory. Inflammation and oxidative stress are two areas where curcumin has shown promise in research.

- **Ginger**: Gingerol, found in ginger, has antioxidant and anti-inflammatory properties. It has the potential to alleviate osteoarthritis and other inflammatory disorders by lowering inflammation.

- **Tomatoes:** Tomatoes Contain Lycopene: Lycopene, found in abundance in tomatoes, is an effective antioxidant with anti-inflammatory characteristics. The bioavailability of lycopene is enhanced when tomatoes are cooked.

- **Oil from olives:** One source of monounsaturated fats and the antioxidant oleocanthal, which has anti-inflammatory properties, is extra virgin olive oil. The anti-inflammatory properties of this food have made it an essential part of the

- **Mediterranean diet:** The anti-inflammatory, antioxidant, and anti-cancer activity of the chemical sulforaphane is found in broccoli.

- **Verdant Tea:**

  •Epigallocatechin gallate (EGCG): Green tea, an antioxidant and anti-inflammatory catechin, is abundant in EGCG.

- **Dark Chocolate:**Flavonoids, which are abundant in high-quality dark chocolate containing a lot of cocoa, can decrease inflammation. Dark chocolate is a good source of these compounds. Consume only a certain amount.

- **Yogurt, kefir, and other fermented foods**: Some studies have shown that the beneficial bacteria found in these foods help reduce inflammation and promote better gut health.

It has been suggested that the anthocyanins contained in cherries, particularly tart cherries, may have anti-inflammatory properties.

Some of the minerals and fiber included in whole grains, such as brown rice, quinoa, and oats, may have an anti-inflammatory effect.

Key Principles of Eating in a Way That Reduces Inflammation

Include a wide variety of foods in your diet to ensure that you are getting the right amount of nutrients.

- **Consume Processed Meals in Moderation**: Reduce your consumption of refined and processed meals, as these foods may be a contributor to inflammation.
- **Hydration:** Consume a large amount of water to promote general health and to assist in the elimination of impurities.

The consumption of these anti-inflammatory foods as part of a diet that is both well-rounded and balanced can make a contribution to a healthier lifestyle and may assist in the management of inflammation inside the body. On the other hand, it is essential to seek the individualized guidance of a healthcare professional, particularly in the event that one is coping with chronic inflammation or other health concerns.

1. **Balanced macronutrients**: Ratio: Aim for a balanced amount of carbohydrates, proteins, and healthy fats. Sources include quinoa, lentils, lean meats, avocados, and olive oil.

   Balanced macronutrients are the appropriate distribution of the three major types of nutrients that provide energy to the body: carbs, proteins, and fats. A balanced macronutrient intake is critical for overall health, vitality, and the appropriate functioning of body processes.

   Below is a breakdown of each macronutrient and its significance in a balanced diet:

❖ **Carbohydrates:**

Carbohydrates have a crucial role in providing energy to the body. They provide glucose, which cells use for a variety of tasks, primarily in the brain and muscles.

Types:

• Simple carbs include glucose, fructose (found in fruits), and sucrose (table sugar).

• Complex carbs are found in starchy meals such as whole grains, legumes, and vegetables.

• Sources include fruits, vegetables, whole grains, legumes, and dairy products.

❖ **Proteins:**

Proteins play a key role in tissue growth, healing, and maintenance. They are composed of amino acids, which are necessary for a variety of physiological functions.

Types:

• Complete proteins, which provide all nine essential amino acids, are sourced from animals and include foods such as meat, fish, eggs, and dairy.

• Plant-based proteins, which can be incomplete due to a lack of a necessary amino acid, are abundant in foods such as beans, lentils, nuts, and seeds.Legumes, nuts, seeds, eggs, dairy, chicken, fish, and plant-based protein sources are some of the sources.

❖ **Fats:**

• Function: Fats play a crucial role in storing energy, making hormones, constructing cells, and absorbing vitamins A, D, E, and K, which are fat-soluble.

Types:

• Animal products, tropical oils, and certain processed foods contain saturated fats. It is advised to consume moderately.

Unsaturated Fats:

• Among the unsaturated fats are the monounsaturated fats that are included in nuts, olive oil, and avocados.

• Included in foods such as walnuts, fatty salmon, flaxseeds, and vegetable oils are polyunsaturated fats.

Sources:

•Avocados, almonds, seeds, fatty fish, olive oil, and plant-based oils are some of the sources.

Achieving Macronutrient Balance:

❖ Calorie Distribution: People's calorie needs are different, but general guidelines suggest getting 45–65% of your calories from carbs, 20–35% from fats, and 10–35% from protein.

❖ Unprocessed, Whole Foods: Eating foods in their natural, unaltered forms helps maintain nutrient balance while cutting back on refined carbs, harmful fats, and added sugars.

Macronutrient requirements differ from one person to the next due to variables including age, sex, degree of physical activity, and health condition. Another factor that might affect the distribution of macronutrients is an individual's goals, such as their weight or their athletic performance.

Knowing the function of each macronutrient, eating a wide variety of nutrient-dense foods, and adjusting the proportions to meet specific needs and objectives are all part of maintaining a healthy diet. Consult with a qualified healthcare provider or registered dietitian to get personalized recommendations based on medical needs and dietary restrictions.

Promoting Good Gut Health

Eating meals that are good for your gut helps keep your digestive system healthy by encouraging the growth and maintenance of good bacteria. Prebiotics, probiotics, and other substances that support gastrointestinal health are commonly found in these foods.

Foods high in fiber, probiotics, and fermented foods (such as kimchi and yogurt) are options.

More information regarding foods that are good for the digestive tract:

❖ **Fruit yoghurt**

Yogurt's probiotics, which include different kinds of good bacteria like Lactobacillus and Bifidobacterium, help keep your digestive tract healthy.

One of the most important minerals for optimum health is calcium, which is abundant in yogurt.

❖ **Probiotic kefir:**

Kefir, a fermented milk drink containing probiotic bacteria, can aid in balancing the microbiota in the gut. Kefir is a great source of protein, vitamins, and minerals.

One example of a fermented food is sauerkraut, which is made from cabbage and is full of beneficial bacteria like Lactobacillus.

Additionally, it provides fiber, which is good for your digestive system, and it's high in fiber.

❖ **Sauerkraut:**

Fermented vegetables, such as cabbage and radishes, are the basis of the Korean dish kimchi, which is rich in probiotics.

It adds variety to the diet thanks to the many spices and flavors it includes.

One traditional Japanese condiment is miso, which is prepared from fermented soybean paste. Soups and stews benefit from their probiotic content.

Nutrient Density: Miso contains minerals and B vitamins that your body needs.

❖ **Tempeh:**

Tempeh is a great way to get plant-based protein and probiotics because it is a fermented soy product.Rich in Nutrients, It's a good source of iron and calcium, among others.

- **Fermented Pickles:** Pickles fermented in brine contain beneficial bacteria and provide a crunchy snack. Low in Calories but may be high in sodium, so moderation is key.

- **Prebiotics:** Bananas contain prebiotics like inulin, which serves as food for beneficial gut bacteria. They are easy to digest and can be a soothing option for the digestive system.

- **Asparagus:** is rich in prebiotics, including inulin, which supports the growth of beneficial bacteria. Nutrient-rich, It provides vitamins, minerals, and antioxidants.

- **Garlic:** contains prebiotics that help nourish beneficial gut bacteria. Garlic has antimicrobial properties that may contribute to a healthy gut.
- **Ginger:** helps maintain a healthy gut lining and reduces inflammation. It's a popular remedy for nausea and gastrointestinal pain.

- **Bone Soup:**
  Collagen, found in bone broth, may help keep the lining of the digestive tract healthy.

- **Hydration:** It supplies water and nutrients that the body needs.

Fundamentals of Gut Health

- **Diversification**: Eat a wide variety of fiber-rich foods and fermented goods to promote a diversified range of microbes and nutrients.
  To prevent getting too much of a certain compound, such as the sodium in pickles, it's best to eat certain items in moderation.
- **Hydration**: For optimal digestive health, drink lots of water.
  Eating foods that are good for your gut can help keep your microbiota in check, which in turn improves your digestion, nutrient absorption, and general health. It is crucial to pay attention to your body and make dietary decisions that are in line with your health objectives because everyone's reactions to these foods are different. See a doctor or certified nutritionist if you have any particular gastrointestinal issues. Keep yourself well hydrated so your cells can work and so your body can eliminate toxins.

  Fruit and herb-infused water, herbal drinks, and plain old water are all on the table.
  Staying properly hydrated is essential for the upkeep of general health and wellness. Staying properly hydrated is critical for sustaining physiological processes, and water is crucial for many of those functions.

The Role of Hydration:

- **Cellular Function**: Cells cannot work correctly without water, which also facilitates important metabolic reactions.
- **Maintaining a Healthy Core Temperature**: Sweating aids in maintaining a healthy core temperature, and staying adequately hydrated is key to rehydrating after exercise.

One important function of water is to facilitate the delivery of nutrients to all parts of the body.Proper hydration aids in keeping joints lubricated, which in turn helps avoid problems like joint stiffness.

How Much Water Should You Drink Every Day?

The National Academies of Sciences, Engineering, and Medicine recommends that males consume approximately 3.7 liters (125 ounces) of water per day and that women consume about 2.7 liters (91 ounces). All foods and drinks that include water are included in this.

• Individual Variation: One's water requirement could change depending on their age, gender, weight, degree of physical activity, and the weather.

Warning Signs of Fluid Loss:

- The body's main signal to drink more is thirst.
- Dark, yellow, or amber urine indicates dehydration.
- The best urine color is pale yellow.
- Dry lips, skin, and mouth indicate dehydration.
- Weakness: Dehydration causes fatigue and energy loss.
- Dizziness and headaches: Not drinking enough water may worsen them.

Considerations for Fluid Needs:

- Increasing physical exertion, especially in hot weather, requires drinking more fluids to replace perspiration.
- Hydration is crucial in hot, humid weather.
- Disease: vomiting, diarrhea, and fever promote fluid loss, requiring more hydration.
- Women who are pregnant or nursing require extra fluids.

Hydration Tips:

- Hydration is best achieved by drinking adequate clean water.
- Drink herbal teas, green tea, infused water, and other beverages to stay hydrated.
- Fruits and vegetables help you keep hydrated because of their high water content,
- Fluid-rich soups and broths can also hydrate.

Electrolytes and Rehydration

When you're really sweating it out or if you're really dehydrated, it may be important to rehydrate by adding more electrolytes (sodium, potassium, chloride).

When electrolyte balance is disturbed, as can happen when someone is sick or loses a lot of fluid, an oral rehydration solution can be helpful.

Drink small amounts of water often during the day instead than gulping down a big glass all at once to stay properly hydrated.

Pay attention to when your body tells you that you're thirsty and act quickly. Light yellow urine is an indication of enough hydration, so be sure to monitor its color.

A person's specific hydration requirements are impacted by their age, weight, and level of physical activity, among other factors.

Optimal health requires doing something as basic as drinking enough water. To maintain good health, it's important to drink plenty of water, sports drinks, and other hydrating fluids on a regular basis and to be aware of the personal aspects that affect water consumption. Drinking enough of water is essential, but everyone has different needs; for specific recommendations, it's best to talk to a doctor.

Staying adequately hydrated is a simple yet fundamental aspect of maintaining optimal health. Regularly consuming a variety of hydrating fluids and being mindful of individual factors that influence hydration needs contribute to overall well-being. It's important to note that individual hydration requirements can vary, and consulting with healthcare professionals can provide personalized guidance.

Mindful Eating

Mindful eating is a practice that encourages a thoughtful and intentional approach to eating, focusing on the sensory experiences, thoughts, and emotions associated with food. This practice aims to promote a healthier relationship with food, enhance the enjoyment of meals, and cultivate awareness of one's eating habits.

Practice: Cultivate awareness during meals to enhance digestion and satisfaction.

Techniques: Chew slowly, savor flavors, and listen to hunger cues.

Here are details about mindful eating:

Awareness of Hunger and Fullness:

- **Listen to Hunger Signals**: Pay attention to physical hunger cues, such as stomach growling, to guide when to eat.
- **Eat Mindfully**: When eating, focus on the experience and sensations of each bite, allowing the body to recognize feelings of fullness.

Engaging the Senses:

- **Savoring Flavors**: Take time to taste and appreciate the flavors of each food. Notice the textures, temperatures, and aromas.
- **Slow Eating**: Chew food slowly and savor each bite. This not only enhances the eating experience but also promotes better digestion.

Mindful Meal Preparation

1. **Practice Mindful Eating by:**
   - **Developing a Bond with Food**: Take part in the act of making food. Feel the flavors, smells, and textures of the ingredients as you prepare them. Be thankful for what you have and the work that went into making it. This will enrich your life.
   - **Emotional Intelligence**: Be Aware of Your Emotions: Keep in mind that feelings like tension, boredom, or sadness might impact your eating patterns.
   - **Mindful Responses**: It's important to think about other methods to deal with and manage emotions besides eating as an unthinking reaction.
2. **Non-Judgmental Awareness**:
   - **Release Guilt:** Approach food choices without judgment or guilt. Acknowledge that all foods can be part of a balanced diet.
   - **Cultivate Self-Compassion**: Be kind and compassionate toward yourself, especially during moments when food choices may not align with ideal preferences.
3. **Eating with Intention:**
   - **Conscious Decision-Making**: Make intentional choices about what to eat based on personal preferences, nutritional needs, and hunger cues.
   - **Mindful Portion Control**: Be aware of portion sizes and choose amounts that satisfy hunger without overeating.
4. **Eliminate Distractions:**
   - **Turn Off Screens**: Minimize distractions such as watching TV or using electronic devices while eating.
   - **Focus on the Meal:** Direct attention solely to the act of eating, creating a more mindful and enjoyable experience.

5. **Mindful Reflection:**
   - **Reflect on Satisfaction**: After finishing a meal, take a moment to reflect on the level of satisfaction and fullness.
   - **Learn from Experiences**: Use reflections to understand personal preferences and adjust eating habits accordingly.
6. **Gratitude Practices**:
   - **Express Gratitude**: Consider expressing gratitude for the food, the hands that prepared it, and the opportunity to nourish the body.
7. **Mindful Hydration**:
   - **Sip Slowly:** Extend mindful eating practices to beverages, such as drinking water slowly and appreciating its refreshing qualities.

Benefits of Mindful Eating

1. **Weight Management**: Mindful eating may contribute to better weight management by promoting awareness of hunger and fullness cues.
2. **Improved Digestion**: Eating slowly and mindfully aids digestion and nutrient absorption.
3. **Enhanced Enjoyment**: By fully engaging with the sensory aspects of food, meals become more satisfying and enjoyable.
4. **Reduced Emotional Eating**: Mindful eating helps break the cycle of emotional eating by fostering awareness of emotional triggers.

Individualized Approach:

- **Recognition**: Acknowledge bio-individuality, understanding that each person's nutritional needs are unique.
- **Personalization**: Tailor the diet to address specific health goals and considerations.

Chapter 12

Healing Diets

A number of healing diets exist, each with its own unique emphasis on what the body needs to thrive generally and on particular health issues. Some well-known healing diets include the following:

- **Mediterranean Eating Plan:**

When you follow the Mediterranean Diet, you take a comprehensive view of your diet, your way of life, and your community. It is important to take into account the overall lifestyle aspects of the Mediterranean way of life, such as frequent physical activity, sharing meals, and a positive attitude toward food satisfaction, in addition to the specific food groups that the diet encourages. If you have any particular health issues, it is imperative that you always seek the advice of healthcare providers or certified dietitians before making any major dietary changes.

Central idea: Packed with healthy ingredients including fresh produce, nuts, seeds, olive oil, and whole grains. Fish and poultry should be consumed in moderation.

Advantages: Good for your heart, reduces inflammation, and has a lot of antioxidants.

Greek, Italian, and Spanish cuisines are the basis for the Mediterranean Diet, which is based on the long-established eating patterns of people living in nations bordering the Mediterranean Sea. A number of chronic disorders have been linked to this diet, and its possible health benefits have just come to light.

Specifics of the Mediterranean Diet are the following:

- **Plant-Based Diet**: A diet rich in fresh produce, whole grains, beans, nuts, and seeds; these foods should form the backbone of a healthy diet.

- **Heart-Healthy Monounsaturated Fats:** Olive oil's main source of fat is olives. Eating nuts and seeds is also recommended.

- **Dairy Moderation**: Consume Greek yogurt and cheese moderately as they are common dairy sources.
- **Protein** should mostly come from fish and seafood, with moderate amounts of eggs Eat just lean red meat.
- Substituting herbs and spices for salt is one way to add flavor to food. The most typical herbs used are rosemary, basil, oregano, and garlic.

Key Foods in the Mediterranean Diet

The Mediterranean Diet is renowned for its health benefits and delicious flavors. Here are some key foods typically included in the Mediterranean Diet

1. Vegetables and Fruits: It is recommended to eat a rainbow of colorful fruits and vegetables, including figs, strawberries, bell peppers, eggplants, zucchini, oranges, and leafy greens.
2. Whole Grains: Bulgur, barley, farro, quinoa, whole grain bread, brown rice, and other whole grains are essential components of the Mediterranean diet because of the fiber, vitamins, and minerals they provide.
3. Legumes: Protein, fiber, and other nutrients abound in legumes including chickpeas, lentils, beans, and peas. Salads, stews, soups, and dips (like hummus) frequently feature them.
4. Nuts and Seeds: Among the many nuts and seeds found in a Mediterranean diet are almonds, walnuts, pistachios, pine nuts, and sesame seeds. Essential nutrients, protein, and good fats are all provided by them.
5. Olive Oil: One of the most essential components of a Mediterranean diet is extra virgin olive oil. In addition to improving food taste, its abundance of monounsaturated fats and antioxidants has many positive effects on health.
6. Seafood & Fish: Heart-healthy omega-3 fatty acids are abundant in fish such as mackerel, sardines, tuna, anchovies, and salmon. Grilled, roasted, or cooked seafood is a common ingredient in many salads.
7. Poultry: The Mediterranean Diet emphasizes moderate consumption of red meat and favors lean protein sources such as chicken and turkey. Common preparations include grilling, roasting, or stewing with them.

8. Dairy: The Mediterranean diet includes moderate consumption of Greek yogurt and cheese, which are good sources of probiotics, protein, and calcium. To make sauces and dips, Greek yogurt is a common ingredient.
9. Herbs and Spices: Garlic, cinnamon, cumin, and paprika are some of the spices and herbs that can be used to add flavor without adding too much sugar or salt. Other herbs and spices include rosemary, thyme, basil, oregano, and garlic.
10. Wine: Red wine is a staple of the Mediterranean diet and, when drunk moderately, is thought to have health benefits owing to its high antioxidant content.

For sustained energy and dietary fiber, incorporate whole grains like brown rice, oats, barley, and

The Mediterranean Diet is based on these foods, which, when coupled with regular physical activity, improve health in all areas.whole wheat into your diet.

Meal Structure:

- **Frequent Meals**: The Mediterranean Diet typically involves three main meals and includes snacks, promoting steady energy levels throughout the day.
- **Family and Social Engagement**: Meals are often enjoyed in a social context, fostering a sense of community and connection.

Health Benefits:

- **Heart Health**: Associated with a reduced risk of cardiovascular diseases due to the emphasis on healthy fats and omega-3 fatty acids.
- **Weight Management**: The diet's focus on whole, nutrient-dense foods and moderate portions may support weight maintenance.
- **Diabetes Prevention**: Linked to a lower risk of type 2 diabetes, potentially due to the diet's impact on insulin sensitivity.
- **Cancer Prevention**: Some studies suggest that the Mediterranean Diet may be associated with a lower risk of certain cancers, although more research is needed.

Cultural and Lifestyle Elements:

- **Physical Activity**: Regular physical activity is often part of the Mediterranean lifestyle, complementing the dietary pattern.
- **Enjoyment of Meals**: The emphasis on savoring and enjoying meals contributes to overall well-being.

Consuming foods that assist decrease inflammation in the body is the main focus of an anti-inflammatory diet. Inflammation is associated with numerous chronic diseases, including heart disease, diabetes, arthritis, and some malignancies. Essential elements of a diet that reduces inflammation include:

The anti-inflammatory diet is designed to reduce inflammation in the body, which is believed to contribute to various chronic diseases. This dietary approach focuses on incorporating foods with anti-inflammatory properties while minimizing the intake of pro-inflammatory foods.

 Here are details about the anti-inflammatory diet:

Emphasis: Foods with anti-inflammatory properties to reduce inflammation.

Inclusions: Fatty fish, berries, leafy greens, nuts, seeds, and turmeric.

Benefits: Alleviates symptoms of inflammation-related conditions.

Anti-Inflammatory Foods:

- **Fruits and Vegetables:** Rich in antioxidants, vitamins, and minerals, fruits and vegetables help combat inflammation. Berries, leafy greens, and cruciferous vegetables are particularly beneficial.
- **Fatty Fish:** Salmon, mackerel, and sardines provide omega-3 fatty acids, known for their anti-inflammatory effects.
- **Nuts and Seeds:** Almonds, walnuts, chia seeds, and flaxseeds are sources of healthy fats and antioxidants.
- **Whole Grains:** Foods like brown rice, quinoa, and oats offer fiber and nutrients with potential anti-inflammatory effects.
- **Healthy Fats:** Olive oil, avocados, and nuts contain monounsaturated fats, which have anti-inflammatory properties.

- **Spices and Herbs**: Anti-inflammatory and antioxidant qualities are well-known for cinnamon, ginger, garlic, and turmeric.

Foods Known to Promote Inflammation:

Certain foods possess anti-inflammatory characteristics, whilst others are recognized for their ability to induce inflammation inside the body. Overindulging in these foods might potentially lead to chronic inflammation, which is associated with a range of health issues. The following foods are recognized for their ability to induce inflammation:

1. Foods containing processed and refined carbohydrates, such as white bread, white rice, pastries, and sugary cereals, have a high glycemic index. This can lead to a rapid increase in blood sugar levels and contribute to inflammation.
2. Sugar and high-fructose corn syrup, commonly included in numerous processed foods and sugary drinks, can lead to inflammation and insulin resistance when consumed as added sugars.
3. Trans fats, commonly present in partially hydrogenated oils utilized in fried foods, processed snacks, margarine, and baked products, have a significant association with inflammation and other chronic illnesses.
4. Saturated fats, when consumed in moderation, may not have negative effects. However, excessive consumption of saturated fats, particularly from sources such as red meat, full-fat dairy products, and some processed meals, can lead to inflammation and cardiovascular disease.
5. Processed meats, including bacon, sausage, hot dogs, and deli meats, are rich in saturated fats, salt, and preservatives. These components can cause inflammation and raise the likelihood of developing chronic diseases.
6. Alcohol: Consuming excessive amounts of alcohol can disturb the balance of bacteria in the gut, escalate inflammation, and compromise the effectiveness of the immune system. Long-term alcohol consumption is linked to a range of inflammatory disorders.

7. Highly processed foods, such as packaged snacks, fast food, frozen meals, and convenience foods, frequently contain harmful fats, refined sugars, and additives that can contribute to inflammation when consumed on a daily basis.

8. Artificial additives, including synthetic tastes, colors, and preservatives like MSG (monosodium glutamate), have the potential to induce inflammation in certain persons.

9. Overconsumption of Omega-6 Fatty Acids: Although omega-6 fatty acids are necessary for good health, taking them excessively compared to omega-3 fatty acids can stimulate inflammation. Omega-6 fatty acids can be found in vegetable oils such as corn, soybean, and sunflower oil.

10. Refined vegetable oils, such as soybean oil, corn oil, and sunflower oil, have significant levels of omega-6 fatty acids. Consuming these oils excessively, particularly when used for frying or in processed meals, might potentially lead to inflammation.

11. Despite regulatory efforts, artificial trans fats can still be found in certain processed and fried meals, which can increase the risk of inflammation and cardiovascular disease.

Restricting the consumption of foods that promote inflammation and prioritizing a diet abundant in whole, minimally processed foods can effectively diminish inflammation and decrease the likelihood of developing chronic diseases.

Processed foods are high in harmful fats, refined sugars, and additives, all of which can exacerbate inflammation.

Anti-Inflammatory Lifestyle Habits

Anti-inflammatory lifestyle habits include engaging in regular physical activity, which has favorable impacts on general health.

- Sufficient Sleep: Inadequate sleep can lead to inflammation, therefore, it is crucial to prioritize excellent sleep habits.

- Stress Management: Prolonged stress can induce inflammation, and activities such as meditation, yoga, and deep breathing can assist in controlling stress levels.
- Engaging in regular physical activity has anti-inflammatory properties and is advantageous for general well-being.
- Sufficient Rest: Inadequate sleep may lead to inflammation, making it crucial to prioritize appropriate sleep habits.
- Stress Management: Prolonged stress can induce inflammation, and activities such as meditation, yoga, and deep breathing can assist in controlling stress levels.

Key Anti-Inflammatory Compounds:

- - Omega-3 Fatty Acids: Omega-3s, present in fatty fish, flaxseeds, and walnuts, exhibit anti-inflammatory properties.
- • Polyphenols are found in abundance in fruits, vegetables, tea, and red wine, and possess antioxidant and anti-inflammatory qualities.
- **Curcumin**: Found in turmeric, curcumin is a potent anti-inflammatory compound.
- **Quercetin:** Present in foods like apples, onions, and berries, quercetin is known for its anti-inflammatory effects.

Meal Planning on an Anti-Inflammatory Diet:

- **Balanced Plate**: Incorporate a variety of colorful fruits and vegetables, lean proteins, healthy fats, and whole grains.
- **Herbs and Spices:** Use turmeric, ginger, garlic, and other anti-inflammatory spices to flavor meals.
- **Hydration:** Stay hydrated with water, herbal teas, and other sugar-free liquids.

Benefits of an Anti-Inflammatory Diet:

• Anti-inflammatory diets may alleviate symptoms of inflammatory diseases like arthritis. • The diet may lower the risk of chronic inflammation-related illnesses like diabetes and heart disease.

• Intestinal health and inflammation are both improved by plant-based diets.

Important Things to Keep in Mind and Seek Expert Advice On

1. **Personal Differences**:

Modifications could be necessary to cater to unique reactions to certain foods. People with preexisting health conditions should consult with doctors or registered dietitians before making significant changes to their diet.

An anti-inflammatory diet consists of eating nutrient-dense, complete foods and incorporating health-promoting lifestyle habits. A healthier, more balanced life is within your reach, even though it won't solve all of your health problems. Because people's demands and responses could vary, it's important to tailor dietary recommendations to each person's unique health situation and objectives.

2. **Plant-Based Diet:**

Fundamentally, it's a plant-based diet that might or might not contain some animal products.

It consists of fruits, vegetables, legumes, nuts, seeds, and whole grains.

Benefits: Increased antioxidants and fiber, and possibly even aid in weight loss.

A plant-based diet consists primarily of plant-based foods with little to no animal products. A lot of people think it's good for the environment and their health.

The following details concern a plant-based diet:

- Fruits and vegetables are the foundation of a plant-based diet, providing vitamins, minerals, fiber, and antioxidants.
- Complete Grains: Whole wheat, quinoa, oats, and brown rice are foods high in additional nutrients and complex carbohydrates.
- Protein: There are several minerals, fiber, and protein inPlant-Based Proteins:
- Legumes: A great source of fiber, protein, and other nutrients are beans, lentils, chickpeas, and peas.
- Tofu and tempeh: These versatile plant-based protein options are made from soy.

- Seitan: A high-protein alternative to meat, seitan is made from wheat gluten.
- Plant-Based Meat Substitutes: A range of plant-based sausages, burgers, and other meat substitutes are available.
- Nuts and Seeds: Provide monounsaturated and polyunsaturated fats, including omega-3 fatty acids.
- Avocado: A nutrient-dense source of monounsaturated fats.
- Olive Oil: A staple in many plant-based diets, offering monounsaturated fats.

Dairy Alternatives:

Dairy substitutes: • Plant-Based Milks: Soy milk, almond milk, oat milk, and other non-dairy substitutes are frequently utilized.

Plant-based yogurts are produced from soy, almond, or coconut, providing alternatives that are free from dairy.

Non-dairy cheese refers to plant-based cheeses crafted using nuts or other plant-derived materials.

Avoiding or Omitting Animal Products:

• Meat: Red meat, chicken, and pork are restricted or omitted.

Some plant-based diets may use fish or seafood occasionally, while others completely exclude them.

• Dairy: Plant-based alternatives are frequently used to substitute dairy products.

Some plant-based diets may eliminate eggs, while others may include them in moderation.

Benefits of a Plant-Based Diet:

- Cardiovascular Health: Studies have associated plant-based diets with a reduced likelihood of developing hypertension, high cholesterol levels, and cardiovascular diseases.
- Plant-based diets, focusing on complete, nutrient-dense foods, can aid in weight management by supporting weight loss and maintenance.

- Plant-based diets can help individuals with type 2 diabetes or those susceptible to the condition achieve improved blood sugar control.
- Plant-based diets with high fiber content promote regular bowel motions and support a healthy digestive tract.
- Environmental Sustainability: Plant-based diets are considered to have a reduced environmental impact compared to animal-based diets due to their lower usage of natural resources and greenhouse gas emissions.

Possible Nutrient Things to Think About

- Vitamin B12: People who eat mostly plants may need to take extra vitamin B12 because it is mostly found in animal products.
- Iron: Non-heme iron from plants is not as easily taken as heme iron from animal sources. It is easier to absorb iron when you eat vitamin C-rich foods with iron-rich plant foods.
- Calcium: Fortified plant milks, tofu, and leafy green veggies are all plant-based sources of calcium.

Balanced Nutrition

Balanced nutrition entails eating a range of foods in proper proportions to sustain health and support bodily processes. A balanced diet should include all of the essential elements, such as carbs, proteins, fats, vitamins, minerals, and water, in the appropriate amounts to fulfill individual needs. Here are some fundamental ideas for balanced nutrition.

1. Macronutrients are nutrients that are required in big quantities, such as carbs, proteins, and lipids.

- Carbohydrates are the body's major source of energy, and they should be obtained mostly from whole grains, fruits, vegetables, and legumes.
- Proteins: Lean meats, chicken, fish, eggs, dairy products, legumes, nuts, and seeds are good sources of protein, which is needed for tissue repair and growth.
- Fats: Healthy fats are essential for cell structure, hormone production, and nutrition uptake. Avocados, almonds, seeds, olive oil, fatty salmon, and flaxseed are also good sources.

2. Micronutrients refer to vital vitamins and minerals that are necessary for various body activities and are needed in lesser amounts.
   - Obtain a diverse array of vitamins, such as vitamins A, C, D, E, K, and B vitamins, by consuming a variety of fruits, vegetables, whole grains, nuts, seeds, and lean proteins.
   - Minerals: Incorporate calcium, magnesium, potassium, iron, zinc, and selenium into your diet by consuming foods such as leafy greens, dairy products, legumes, nuts, seeds, and lean meats.
3. Dietary fiber: Constipation, proper blood sugar regulation, and digestive health all depend on getting enough dietary fiber. There is a lot of fiber in whole foods including nuts, seeds, fruits, and vegetables.
4. Fluids: Water plays an essential role in keeping the body hydrated, controlling core temperature, and facilitating a number of metabolic functions. Aim for a glass of water every hour of the day and be sure to eat enough of water-rich produce.
5. Eating moderately a diverse range of foods will guarantee that you get all the nutrients your body needs. A balanced diet requires moderation since eating too much of any one food, no matter how healthy, can throw off the balance.

Plant-Based Lifestyle

• More Than Just a Diet, a plant-based lifestyle usually includes more than just food. It can also include ethical concerns, sustainable living, and general health.

When you switch to a plant-based diet, you choose to eat more foods that come from plants. You can change your diet to fit your tastes and nutritional needs. Health care experts or registered dietitians can give you personalized advice on how to start and stick to a plant-based diet while still meeting your nutritional needs.

1. **Paleolithic (Paleo) Diet:**

Concept: Mimics the presumed diet of Paleolithic humans, emphasizing whole foods.

Inclusions: Lean meats, fish, fruits, vegetables, nuts, and seeds.

Benefits: Supports weight loss, improved blood sugar control.

The Paleolithic diet, often referred to as the Paleo diet, is a dietary approach that attempts to mimic the presumed diet of Paleolithic humans, dating back to the Stone Age. The underlying principle is to focus on whole, unprocessed foods that our ancestors might have consumed. Here are details about the Paleo diet:

Focus on Whole Foods:

- **Lean Proteins**: Emphasis on animal proteins such as meat, poultry, fish, and eggs. These provide essential amino acids and important nutrients.
- **Fruits and Vegetables**: Rich sources of vitamins, minerals, fiber, and antioxidants. A variety of colorful produce is encouraged.
- **Nuts and seeds** are a great source of protein, healthy fats, and minerals. Common choices include of chia seeds, flaxseeds, walnuts, and almonds.
- **Grains**: Grains like rice, oats, and wheat are not part of this category. Getting your carbs from veggies and fruits is the way to go.
- Legumes: Due to their high quantities of lectin and phytic acid, legumes including peanuts, beans, and lentils are not included.
- When you have issues with lactose or casein, it's best to stay away from dairy products like cheese, yogurt, and milk.
- Processed Foods: Foods that have been through a lot of processing, refined sugar, or artificial ingredients are not allowed on this diet.

Healthy Fats:

- **Natural Fats**: Encourages the consumption of natural fats, including those from avocados, nuts, seeds, and olive oil.
- **Omega-3 Fatty Acids**: Fatty fish like salmon, mackerel, and sardines are recommended for their omega-3 fatty acids.

Limitation of Certain Cooking Methods:

- **Preferable Cooking Methods:** Advocates for cooking methods such as grilling, baking, steaming, and sautéing, while discouraging deep-frying.

Emphasis on Grass-Fed and Pasture-Raised:

- **Meat Quality**: Encourages the consumption of grass-fed and pasture-raised meats to enhance the nutrient profile and omega-3 fatty acid content.

Nutrient Density:

- **Focus on Nutrient-Rich Foods**: The emphasis is on consuming foods that are nutrient-dense, providing a range of essential vitamins and minerals.

Hydration:

- **Water**: Encourages regular water consumption for hydration.

Physical Activity:

- **Active Lifestyle**: Often promotes an active lifestyle, aligning with the presumed physical activity levels of our ancestors.

Potential Benefits:

- **Weight Management**: Some individuals may experience weight loss due to the emphasis on whole foods and the exclusion of processed foods.
- **Blood Sugar Control**: The diet's focus on whole, unprocessed foods may contribute to better blood sugar control.

- **Improved Lipid Profiles**: Some studies suggest potential improvements in lipid profiles, including lower levels of triglycerides and increased levels of HDL cholesterol.

Considerations and Criticisms:

- **Nutrient Imbalances**: Critics argue that the exclusion of entire food groups may lead to nutrient imbalances.
- **Sustainability**: The sustainability of a strict Paleo diet has been questioned, especially due to potential environmental concerns associated with increased meat consumption.
- **Individual Variation**: Responses to the Paleo diet can vary, and it may not be suitable for everyone.

Individualization and Moderation:

- **Flexibility:** Some individuals choose a more flexible approach, incorporating certain foods like dairy or legumes based on individual preferences and tolerances.
- **Balanced Nutrient Intake**: It's important to pay attention to individual nutrient needs and ensure a balanced intake of essential nutrients.

Following a Paleo diet means transitioning to whole, unprocessed foods, focusing on lean proteins, fruits, vegetables, nuts, and seeds. It is crucial to take into account individual health objectives, dietary requirements, and tolerances when following any diet. Seeking advice from healthcare specialists or certified dietitians can offer personalized recommendations on the compatibility of the Paleo diet with particular health needs.

Whole30

Whole30 is a dietary regimen that aims to reset your eating patterns, eliminate potentially inflammatory foods, and enhance general health. It includes a 30-day elimination phase in which participants avoid dietary groups that are thought to be potentially hazardous or problematic for some people.

Whole30 is a 30-day regimen that excludes specific foods to pinpoint potential sensitivities.

- ❖ Exclusions: Sugar, wheat, dairy, legumes, and processed foods.
- ❖ Advantages: Resets dietary patterns, pinpoints food triggers.

The Whole30 program is a month-long nutritional reset plan that aims to assist individuals in identifying and removing potentially troublesome foods from their diet, enabling them to understand the impact of various foods on their health and well-being. Here are specifics regarding the Whole30 program:

❖ **Exclusion of Certain Foods:**

• Sugar and Sweeteners: Any type of added sugar, whether natural or artificial, is not allowed.

• Grains such as wheat, rice, oats, corn, and others are removed.

Legumes such as beans, lentils, peanuts, and soy products are limited.

• Dairy: All dairy items such as milk, cheese, and yogurt are not allowed.

• Processed Foods: All processed foods, additives, and artificial components are removed.

• Alcohol: Prohibition of alcoholic beverages.

• Specific food additives like carrageenan, MSG, and sulfites are not used.

Whole, unprocessed foods:

• Meat and Seafood: Comprises a range of meats, poultry, and seafood, ideally in their intact and unaltered states.

• All veggies are permitted, encouraging a varied consumption of colorful and nutrient-rich choices.

• Fresh fruits are recommended but should be consumed in moderation because of their inherent sugar content.

• Nuts and Seeds: Consume in restricted to moderate quantities.

• Permissible Healthy Fats: Healthy fats from sources such as avocados, olive oil, and coconut oil are allowed.

• Sweeteners and Sugar: No additional sugar, either natural or artificial, is allowed.

• Grains: Corn, wheat, oats, and rice are all off-limits.

• Legumes: Restricted items include peanuts, beans, lentils, and soy.

Milk, cheese, and yoghurt are all considered dairy products, but there are others that aren't.

• Foods that have been processed: We rid our diet of all processed foods, additives, and artificial components.

You are not allowed to have any alcoholic beverages.

• Some Food Additives: Things like sulfites, carrageenan, and monosodium glutamate are not used.

Whole, Unprocessed Foods:

Included in this category are many types of meat, poultry, and shellfish, ideally in their natural, uncooked states.

• Vegetables: Any kind of vegetable is fair game, so you can eat a rainbow of health benefits.

Because of their natural sugar content, fresh fruits should be enjoyed in moderation, although they are still highly encouraged.

Moderate consumption of nuts and seeds is recommended.

It is acceptable to consume healthy fats derived from avocados, olive oil, and coconut oil.

No Tracking or Counting:

- **Emphasis on Whole Foods**: Instead of counting calories or macros, the focus is on consuming whole, nutrient-dense foods.

Commitment to the 30-Day Duration:

- **Strict Adherence:** The program encourages strict adherence to the guidelines for the entire 30-day period to allow the body to reset and to accurately assess the impact of specific foods.

Reintroduction Phase:

- **Gradual Reintroduction:** After completing the 30 days, participants systematically reintroduce eliminated foods one at a time to observe how each food group affects their body.
- **Observing Reactions:** This phase helps identify potential sensitivities or reactions to specific foods.

Focus on Non-Scale Victories:

- **Non-Weight Benefits**: The program emphasizes the potential non-scale victories, such as improved energy, sleep, digestion, and mental clarity, rather than solely focusing on weight loss.

No Cheat Days:

- **Strict Adherence:** Participants are encouraged to avoid any deviations or cheat days during the 30-day period to experience the full benefits of the program.

Education and Support:

- **Resources:** The Whole30 program provides resources, including a comprehensive website, books, and social media communities, to support participants throughout the process.
- **Community:** Participants can connect with others following the program for guidance, encouragement, and shared experiences.

Post-program mindset involves promoting attentive and informed food choices beyond the 30-day program.

The Whole30 program is designed as a temporary reset rather than a permanent diet. The goal is to assist individuals in recognizing possible food sensitivities, enhancing overall well-being, and developing a healthier connection with food. It is recommended to get advice from healthcare specialists or registered dietitians when following a nutritional program, particularly if you have certain health issues or dietary requirements.

Ayurvedic Diet:

The Ayurvedic diet is based on Ayurveda, an ancient medical system that started in India more than 3,000 years ago. This comprehensive health method focuses on achieving equilibrium and unity among the body, mind, and spirit.

Follows Ayurvedic principles by tailoring nutrition to specific doshas (body kinds).

The elements include six tastes: sweet, sour, salty, bitter, pungent, and astringent.

Advantages: Harmonizes doshas, promotes general health.

The Ayurvedic diet is customized based on each individual's specific constitution, referred to as their "dosha." Three main doshas are Vata, Pitta, and Kapha. Here are specifics on the Ayurvedic diet:

Comprehending Doshas:

- ❖ Vata: Pertaining to the elements air and space, Vata is distinguished by attributes of aridity, low temperature, airiness, and motion.
- ❖ Pitta, which is associated with the elements fire and water, possesses the attributes of heat, intensity, acuity, and metamorphosis.
- ❖ Kapha: Affiliated with the earth and water elements, Kapha is distinguished by its weight, sluggishness, chill, and stability.

Harmonizing Doshas:

- ❖ Tailored Approach: The Ayurvedic diet is customized to suit the specific dosha or dosha combination of an individual.
- ❖ Achieving Equilibrium: The objective is to harmonize the intrinsic attributes of every dosha through the integration of foods possessing contrasting qualities.

Six Tastes (Rasas):

- **Sweet (Madhura):** Nourishes and soothes. Examples include whole grains, dairy, and sweet fruits.
- **Sour (Amla):** Stimulates digestion. Examples include citrus fruits, yogurt, and fermented foods.
- **Salty (Lavana):** Enhances flavor and moistens. Examples include sea salt and certain vegetables.

- **Bitter (Tikta):** Detoxifies and cools. Examples include leafy greens, turmeric, and bitter melon.
- **Pungent (Katu):** Stimulates digestion and metabolism. Examples include spicy foods, ginger, and garlic.
- **Astringent (Kashaya):** Contracts tissues and dries. Examples include legumes, green apples, and pomegranates.

Seasonal Eating:

- **Harmonizing with Nature**: The Ayurvedic diet emphasizes eating seasonally to align with the qualities of the current season and maintain balance.

Favoring Whole, Fresh Foods:

- **Minimizing Processed Foods:** The diet encourages the consumption of whole, fresh foods over processed and refined options.

Individualized Meal Plans:

- **Dietary Adjustments:** Depending on an individual's dosha, dietary adjustments may be made to balance excesses or deficiencies.

Herbs and Spices:

- **Therapeutic Use:** Herbs and spices are often used for their therapeutic properties. For example, turmeric is anti-inflammatory, and ginger aids digestion.

Mindful Eating Practices:

Ayurvedic eating principles incorporate mindful practices, which involve cultivating a state of presence during meals and attentively recognizing signals of hunger and satiety—all of which contribute to the establishment of a mind-body connection:

Pairing Foods:

In order to promote digestive harmony and prevent the accumulation of contradictory qualities, the Ayurvedic diet prescribes particular food combinations that aid digestion.

Warm water or herbal teas are frequently favored over frigid beverages for their ability to aid

Consistent Daily Path (Dinacharya):

A well-rounded way of life encompasses more than just the Ayurvedic diet; it consists of daily practices and routines that are intended to foster holistic health.

One of the main goals of Ayurvedic practice is promoting healthy digestion.

- Harmonious Energy: When people strive to live in harmony with their dosha, they want to keep their energy levels balanced and their vitality high.
- One goal of the Ayurvedic diet is to help people achieve a state of mental and physical balance.

Advice from Ayurvedic Experts:

For a more customized approach, people can seek out Ayurvedic practitioners to find out their dosha and get nutritional advice that are specifically suited to them.

Keep in mind that the Ayurvedic diet is more of a system, and that people react differently to it. An individual's distinct constitution and health objectives can inform the individualized advice provided by consultations with trained Ayurvedic practitioners. Furthermore, people should see healthcare providers for guidance with particular health issues.

The Syndrome of Gut and Psychology, or GAPS Food Plan

Objective: Addresses mental health difficulties by focusing on gut health.

The first step is to ease back into eating solid foods, with a focus on fermented foods and bone broth. Helps with digestion and could even have a positive effect on mental health.

Dr. Natasha Campbell-McBride created the GAPS (Gut and Psychology Syndrome) diet as a therapeutic dietary strategy to treat and alleviate gut-related problems, especially those that are thought to be associated with neurological and psychological disorders. As part of the GAPS treatment, which also involves targeted nutrition and lifestyle adjustments, the diet is frequently utilized. Knowledge regarding the GAPS diet can be found here:

Focus on Gut Health:

- **Leaky Gut Theory**: The GAPS diet is based on the concept of "leaky gut," suggesting that an impaired gut lining contributes to the development of various health issues, including psychological and neurological conditions.

Elimination and Introduction Phases:

- **Introduction Phase**: Initially, the diet involves an introduction phase that includes easily digestible foods to soothe the gut lining. This phase progresses through stages with the gradual addition of more complex foods.
- **Full GAPS Diet:** After the introduction phase, individuals move to the full GAPS diet, which includes a broader range of foods but continues to exclude certain items.

Part of the GAPS Diet is bone broth, which is high in nutrients and thought to aid in gut repair.

Consuming fermented foods such as sauerkraut, kimchi, yogurt, and kefir can help maintain a balanced population of beneficial bacteria in the digestive tract.

Protein-rich meats and seafood that are organic and of high quality are part of the package.

The use of good fats, such as those found in animal products, olive oil, and coconut oil, is highly encouraged.

The majority of vegetables that are not starchy are OK.

As a first step in the diet, you may be asked to cut back on fruit, especially fruits that are high in sugar. Oftentimes, berries are suggested.

Foods Excluded or Limited:

- **Grains:** Grains, including wheat, oats, and rice, are typically eliminated.
- **Processed Foods:** Highly processed foods, sugars, and artificial additives are restricted.
- **Certain Dairy:** During the introduction phase, dairy is limited to fermented dairy products. Later, some individuals may reintroduce properly prepared dairy.
- **Starchy Vegetables**: Initially, starchy vegetables may be limited. They are gradually reintroduced as tolerated.

Emphasis on Nutrient Density:

- **Nourishing Foods**: The diet emphasizes nutrient-dense foods to support overall health and healing.

Supplements and lifestyle factors:
• Certain supplements, such as probiotics and fish oil, may be advised based on individual needs.
• The GAPS protocol recommends lifestyle changes, such as stress management, sleep, and physical activity.

Individualized Approach:
• The GAPS diet is customized to address individual health challenges, sensitivities, and responses.
Potential benefits:
• The diet promotes gut repair and may help treat gut dysbiosis.
• Promoting gut health may benefit psychological and neurological disorders, according to advocates.

Points to Think About: • Speak with Practitioners: People who are interested in the GAPS diet frequently speak with medical professionals or other practitioners who are knowledgeable about the protocol.

• Potential for Nutrient Gaps: Careful preparation may be necessary to prevent nutrient deficits during the diet, especially during its restricted phases.

Time and Observation:

❖ Individual Progress: The length of the GAPS diet varies according to each person's requirements and level of development. Some people might stick to the regimen for several months or even longer.

❖ Monitoring Response: To determine whether a diet is helpful, it is imperative to regularly check symptoms and overall health.

People who are thinking about starting the GAPS diet should speak with healthcare providers, just like with any therapeutic diet, especially if they have any underlying health issues. The GAPS diet is not well recognized, and the scientific and medical sectors are still debating whether or not it is effective for treating particular ailments.

Ketogenic Diet

The ketogenic diet, or keto for short, is an eating plan that aims to put the body into a metabolic state of ketosis by reducing carbohydrate intake and increasing fat consumption. Ketosis is characterized by a metabolic shift away from glucose and toward ketones, which are byproducts of fatty acid breakdown.

Specifics of the ketogenic diet are as follows:

- The Mechanism of the Ketogenic Diet: A Low-Carbohydrate, High-Fat Diet That Induces Ketosis for Energy.

- Edibles: Avocados, extra-virgin olive oil, fatty seafood, and veggies that aren't starchy.

- Gains: Less body fat, sharpe's mind.

Essential Nutrient Ratios:

• Heavy Fat: Healthful fats make up a large portion of the diet, usually between 70 and 80 percent of the calories consumed each day.

• Moderate Protein Intake: Protein accounts for about 20-25% of total calories consumed each day.

• Carbohydrate Restriction: Carbohydrates should not make up more than 5-10% of your daily calorie intake.

Typical Items on a Ketogenic Diet: • Heart-Healthy Fats: Avocado, coconut, olive, butter, ghee, and fatty seafood are staples.

Meat, fowl, shellfish, eggs, and some dairy products are good sources of protein.

• Non-Starchy veggies: When consumed in moderation, low-carb veggies such as broccoli, zucchini, cauliflower, and leafy greens are acceptable.

• Seeds and Nuts: Included for protein and healthy fats are flaxseeds, chia seeds, walnuts, and almonds.

Monitoring Ketosis

Restricted or Not Allowed Foods:

Because of their high carbohydrate content, you are banned from eating grains, legumes, starchy veggies, and the majority of fruits.

Processed sweets, honey, and sweeteners with a lot of carbohydrates should be avoided.

• Meals that have been processed: Eat as few processed and refined meals as possible.

• Some Dairy: There aren't many high-carb dairy products, and some people prefer full-fat varieties.

Entering the Ketosis State:

• Depleting Glycogen reserves: At the outset, the body begins to produce ketones from fats when its glycogen reserves are depleted.

During the adaptation period, which can last anywhere from a few days to a few weeks, people may feel what is commonly known as the "keto flu," a fleeting combination of symptoms that can include things like headaches, irritability, and exhaustion.

Factors to Consider and Obstacles to Overcome

* Nutrient Intake: It is critical to maintain a sufficient consumption of vital nutrients, including vitamins and minerals, due to the restriction of certain dietary groups.
* Sustainability: The restrictive nature of the ketogenic diet may pose a challenge for certain individuals in terms of its long-term viability.
* Variability among Individuals: The efficacy of the ketogenic diet may differ, and not all individuals may perceive identical advantages.

Cyclical or Keto-targeted Diets:

The Cyclical Ketogenic Diet (CKD) consists of alternating days of intense ketosis and days with an increased carbohydrate intake.A targeted carbohydrate intake is permitted during a targeted ketogenic diet (TKD) in order to enhance physical performance during exercises.

Medical Supervision:

• Pregnancy: Prior to commencing a ketogenic diet, individuals with specific medical conditions, including liver disease or pancreatitis, ought to consult with a healthcare professional.

* Long-Term Monitoring: Healthcare professionals should oversee long-term adherence to the ketogenic diet in order to verify its impact on overall health and well-being.
* It is advisable for individuals contemplating the ketogenic diet to seek guidance from healthcare professionals or registered dietitians, particularly if they have preexisting health conditions or concerns, as with any substantial dietary alteration. Due to the

fact that the ketogenic diet may not be appropriate for all individuals, its potential benefits and drawbacks must be thoroughly assessed in a personalized setting.

- Preexisting Conditions: People with specific medical issues, like pancreatitis or liver disease, should consult a doctor before beginning a ketogenic diet.
- Long-Term Monitoring: Healthcare providers should keep tabs on patients' long-term ketogenic diet adherence to make sure they're healthy overall.

Anyone thinking about going on the ketogenic diet should talk to their doctor or a certified dietitian before making any major changes to their eating habits, particularly if they have any preexisting health issues. Every person's unique circumstances call for a thorough assessment of the pros and cons of the ketogenic diet, since it might not be right for them.

Low-FODMAP Diet

An helpful technique for controlling symptoms of irritable bowel syndrome (IBS) is the low-FODMAP diet. To guarantee nutritional adequacy and customized counsel, however, its implementation should be overseen by healthcare specialists, particularly qualified dietitians. The Low-FODMAP diet isn't right for everyone, so it's important to talk to doctors before starting it. They can help you stick to it and keep it under control in the long run.

Low-FODMAP Diet Phases:

- **Elimination Phase**: Initially, individuals follow a strict low-FODMAP diet to reduce symptoms. This phase typically lasts 2-6 weeks.
- **Reintroduction Phase**: FODMAP-containing foods are systematically reintroduced to identify specific triggers. This phase helps identify which FODMAPs can be tolerated and in what amounts.
- **Personalization Phase**: Based on individual responses, a personalized and sustainable diet is developed.

Foods Included and Restricted:

- **Low-FODMAP Foods**: Includes certain fruits (e.g., berries, citrus), vegetables (e.g., spinach, carrots), proteins (e.g., meat, fish), and some grains (e.g., rice, oats).
- **High-FODMAP Foods:** Restricted during the elimination phase and include certain fruits (e.g., apples, cherries), vegetables (e.g., onions, garlic), dairy products, and specific grains and legumes.

Common High-FODMAP Foods:

- Fruits: Apples, pears, watermelon, mango.

- Vegetables: Onions, garlic, asparagus, cauliflower.

- Legumes: Beans, lentils, chickpeas.

- Dairy: Milk, yogurt, soft cheeses.

- Sweeteners: Honey, high-fructose corn syrup, certain sugar alcohols.

FODMAP-Friendly Cooking and Substitutions:

- FODMAP-Friendly Ingredients: Use FODMAP-friendly alternatives, such as garlic-infused oil instead of garlic or green onions instead of regular onions.

- Portion Control: Some high-FODMAP foods may be tolerated in smaller portions.

Benefits and Management of Symptoms:

- Symptom Reduction: The Low-FODMAP diet aims to reduce symptoms associated with IBS, such as bloating, gas, abdominal pain, and changes in bowel habits.

- Individualized Approach: The reintroduction phase allows for personalization, as not all individuals have the same triggers.

Things to Think About When Eating: • Dietitian Oversight: For optimal nutritional status and to avoid nutrient shortages, it is recommended to follow the Low-FODMAP diet in the company of a certified nutritionist.

Upkeep Over Time:

Individuals move from the reintroduction phase to a varied diet after which they avoid particular high-FODMAP triggers.

Possible Negative Effects:

• The Diet Can Be Strict, Restricting Access To Some Nutrient-Dense Foods.

• Personal Reactions: Some people have varying reactions to FODMAPs, and a low-FODMAP diet may not be necessary or helpful for all irritable bowel syndrome (IBS) sufferers.

DASH (Dietary Approaches to Stop Hypertension) Diet

The DASH diet (Dietary Approaches to Stop Hypertension) is a dietary strategy that aims to prevent and control hypertension (high blood pressure). It stresses a balanced and heart-healthy diet, with a focus on nutrient-dense foods that promote overall cardiovascular health. Here are some specifics regarding the DASH diet:

To regulate blood pressure, focus on fruits, vegetables, lean meats, and low-fat dairy products.

Whole grains, nuts, and seeds are all recommended, as is a low salt intake.
Benefits: Promotes heart health and regulates blood pressure.

Individual nutritional needs vary, so speak with a healthcare practitioner or qualified dietitian before making significant dietary adjustments. These healing diets are generic guidelines that can be modified based on individual health objectives and circumstances.

Limitation of Sodium:

- **Reduced Sodium Intake**: Emphasizes the importance of reducing sodium intake to help control blood pressure. This involves limiting the consumption of high-sodium processed foods.

Moderate Alcohol Consumption:

Limited Alcohol Intake: Recommends moderation in alcohol consumption, suggesting up to one drink per day for women and up to two drinks per day for men.

Portion Control:

- **Balanced Portions**: Encourages mindful eating and portion control to help maintain a healthy weight.

Rich in Potassium, Magnesium, and Calcium:

- **Potassium**: High-potassium foods like bananas, oranges, and leafy greens are emphasized for their potential to counteract the effects of sodium on blood pressure.
- **Magnesium**: Foods rich in magnesium, such as nuts, seeds, and whole grains, are included.
- **Calcium:** Low-fat or fat-free dairy products provide a source of calcium for bone health.

Adaptable to Individual Needs:

- **Flexibility**: The DASH diet is adaptable and can be adjusted based on individual dietary preferences and health conditions.

Meal Planning and Recipes:

- **Guidance:** Provides guidance on meal planning and offers recipes to help individuals incorporate DASH principles into their daily eating habits.

Evidence-Based Approach:

- **Research Support**: The DASH diet is supported by extensive scientific research, including studies demonstrating its effectiveness in lowering blood pressure.

Potential Benefits:

- **Blood Pressure Control**: The primary goal of the DASH diet is to help prevent and manage hypertension.

- **Cardiovascular Health**: The emphasis on whole, nutrient-dense foods contributes to overall cardiovascular health.
- **Weight Management**: The DASH diet, with its focus on balanced nutrition, may support weight management.

Long-Term Lifestyle Approach:

- **Sustainability:** Designed as a long-term lifestyle approach, the DASH diet promotes sustainable changes rather than short-term restrictions.

The DASH diet is often recommended by healthcare professionals for individuals looking to manage or prevent hypertension. It aligns with broader guidelines for heart-healthy eating and provides a practical framework for adopting a balanced and nutrient-rich diet. Before making significant changes to dietary habits, individuals should consult with healthcare professionals or registered dietitians, especially those with existing health conditions or specific dietary needs.

Chapter 13

Natural Remedies for Allergies

Although some people find relief from their allergy symptoms with natural remedies, it's crucial to remember that they shouldn't be used in place of guidance from a medical practitioner. Seek advice from a medical expert before attempting any home cures if you suffer from serious allergies or are already on medication. Some people get relief from their allergy symptoms by using the following natural remedies:

❖ **Local Honey**: Consuming raw, local honey may help desensitize your body to pollen allergens over time. Bees collect pollen from local plants, and consuming small amounts of this pollen through honey may help build immunity.

❖ **Quercetin:** Quercetin is a natural flavonoid found in many fruits, vegetables, and herbs. It has anti-inflammatory and antihistamine properties, which can help reduce allergy symptoms. Foods rich in quercetin include apples, onions, kale, and citrus fruits. Quercetin supplements are also available.

❖ **Nettle Leaf**: Nettle leaf (Urtica dioica) has natural antihistamine properties and can help relieve allergy symptoms such as sneezing, itching, and congestion. Nettle leaf can be consumed as a tea or taken in supplement form.

❖ **Butterbur:** Butterbur (Petasites hybridus) is an herb that has been shown to relieve allergy symptoms, particularly nasal congestion and hay fever. It works as a natural antihistamine and anti-inflammatory. Look for butterbur supplements standardized to remove pyrrolizidine alkaloids, which can be harmful.

❖ **Probiotics:** Probiotics are beneficial bacteria that support immune function and may help reduce allergic reactions. Consuming probiotic-rich foods such as yogurt, kefir, sauerkraut, and kimchi, or taking probiotic supplements, can help balance gut flora and support overall immune health.

- ❖ **Local Bee Pollen**: Similar to local honey, consuming small amounts of local bee pollen may help desensitize your body to pollen allergens. Start with small amounts to ensure you don't have any adverse reactions.

- ❖ **Essential Oils:** Some essential oils, such as peppermint, eucalyptus, and lavender, have natural anti-inflammatory and decongestant properties that can help relieve allergy symptoms. Diffuse these oils in your home or dilute them with a carrier oil and apply them topically.

- ❖ **Saline Nasal Rinse:** Using a saline nasal rinse can help clear nasal passages and reduce congestion by flushing out allergens and irritants..

- ❖ **Turmeric**: Adding turmeric to your diet or taking curcumin supplements may help reduce inflammation and alleviate allergy symptoms. Turmeric contains curcumin, a compound with potent anti-inflammatory properties.

- ❖ **Avoid Allergen Triggers**: While natural remedies can help manage allergy symptoms, it's essential to minimize exposure to allergens that trigger your symptoms

Chapter14

Home Herbal Toolkit

Creating a home herbal toolkit can be a great way to have natural remedies readily available for common health concerns. Here's a suggested list of herbs and herbal products to include in your toolkit, along with their potential uses:

1. Aloe Vera Gel: Soothes minor burns, cuts, and skin irritations.
2. Calendula Cream or Salve: Promotes wound healing and soothes skin irritations.
3. Echinacea Tincture or Capsules: Supports immune function and helps fight off colds and flu.
4. Peppermint Essential Oil: Relieves headaches, nausea, and digestive discomfort; also used for aromatherapy.
5. Lavender Essential Oil: Promotes relaxation, relieves stress and anxiety, and soothes skin irritations.
6. Chamomile Tea Bags: Calms nerves, promotes relaxation, aids digestion, and relieves menstrual cramps.
7. Ginger Tea Bags or Ginger Capsules: Relieves nausea, aids digestion, and reduces inflammation.
8. Eucalyptus Essential Oil: Clears congestion, relieves respiratory symptoms, and repels insects.
9. Arnica Gel or Cream: Reduces inflammation, relieves muscle aches and pains, and promotes healing of bruises and sprains.
10. Honey: Soothes sore throats, boosts immunity, and can be used in homemade remedies.
11. Apple Cider Vinegar: Aids digestion, supports immune function, and can be used topically for skin conditions.
12. Olive Leaf Extract: Supports immune function, reduces inflammation, and may help with colds and flu.

13. Turmeric Capsules or Powder: Reduces inflammation, supports joint health, and boosts immunity.

14. Garlic Capsules or Raw Garlic: Boosts immune function, supports cardiovascular health, and has antimicrobial properties.

15. Nettle Leaf Tea: Relieves allergy symptoms, supports kidney function, and provides essential nutrients.

16. St. John's Wort Oil or Tincture: Relieves nerve pain, soothes skin irritations, and supports emotional well-being.

17. White Willow Bark Capsules: Relieves pain and inflammation, particularly headaches and muscle aches.

18. Valerian Root Tincture or Capsules: Promotes relaxation, relieves insomnia, and reduces anxiety.

19. Dandelion Root Tea or Capsules: Supports liver health, aids digestion, and acts as a diuretic.

20. Ginseng Capsules: Increases energy and vitality, supports adrenal health, and boosts immune function.

Chapter 15

Herbs And Their Uses

Herbal treatments have been used for generations to treat a wide range of common disorders, offering natural alternatives for people seeking holistic approaches to wellness. While major health concerns should be addressed by a healthcare expert, herbal remedies can effectively handle many minor health conditions. Here's an in-depth look at herbal cures for common diseases.

1. **Peppermint (Mentha piperita**) can help with digestive issues.

    Properties: antispasmodic and carminative.

    Uses: Reduces indigestion, bloating, and gas. Peppermint tea and pills are often utilized.

2. **Ginger (zingiber officinale):**

    Properties: anti-inflammatory and digestive.

    Uses: Reduces nausea, motion sickness, and improves digestion. Fresh ginger tea or ginger pills may be effective.

3. **Respiratory Congestion: Eucalyptus (Eucalyptus globulus)**

    Properties: Decongestant and antibacterial.

    Uses: Clears respiratory passageways and relieves congestion. It is typical to inhale eucalyptus steam or use eucalyptus oil diffusers.

4. **Thyme (Thymus vulgaris**).

    Properties: antimicrobial and expectorant.

    Uses: Promotes respiratory health and helps remove mucus. Thyme tea or thyme-infused honey may be useful.

5. **Licorice root (Glycyrrhiza glabra**) is known for its soothing and expectorant properties.

Uses: Reduces throat discomfort and supports healthy mucus production. Licorice tea and lozenges are common options.

6. **Sleep Disorders: Valerian (Valeriana officinali**s):

Properties: sedative and soothing.

Uses: Promotes relaxation and better sleep. Valerian tea and valerian root capsules are common medicines.

7. **Lavender (Lavandula angustifolia):**

Properties: Relaxing, mild sedative.

Uses: Promotes calmness and relaxation. Lavender-infused pillows, sachets, or essential oil diffusion are popular methods.

8. **Chamomile (Matricaria chamomilla):**

Properties: Calming, sedative.

Uses: Induces sleep, reduces anxiety. Chamomile tea or chamomile essential oil in a diffuser can be effective.

9. Stress and Anxiety**: Ashwagandha (Withania somnifera**):

Properties: Adaptogenic, calming.

Uses: Helps the body adapt to stress, reduces anxiety. Ashwagandha capsules or powdered root are common choices.

10. **Passionflower (Passiflora incarnata):**

Properties: Sedative, nervine.

Uses: Calms the nervous system, reduces anxiety. Passionflower tea or tincture can be beneficial.

11. **Lemon Balm (Melissa officinalis):**

Properties: Calming, uplifting.

Uses: Eases nervous tension, promotes relaxation. Lemon balm tea or essential oil diffusion is common.

12. **Turmeric (Curcuma longa**): Joint Pain and Inflammation

Properties: Anti-inflammatory, analgesic.

Uses: Reduces joint inflammation, alleviates pain. Turmeric capsules or turmeric-infused dishes are popular choices.

13. **Devil's Claw (Harpagophytum procumbens):**

Properties: Anti-inflammatory, analgesic.

Uses: Eases arthritis pain, reduces inflammation. Devil's Claw capsules or tinctures are common.

14. **Ginger (Zingiber officinale):**

Properties: Anti-inflammatory, analgesic.

Uses: Aids in reducing joint pain and inflammation. Fresh ginger tea or ginger capsules can be beneficial.

15. **Feverfew (Tanacetum parthenium) for headaches:**

Properties: reduces inflammation and widens blood vessels.

Uses: Lowers the number and severity of headaches. You can take feverfew pills or eat fresh leaves.

16. **Calendula (Calendula officinalis**): Itchy Skin

Properties: reduces inflammation and soothes the skin.

Uses: Helps wounds heal and calms skin irritations. You can put calendula-infused oil or cream on your skin.

17. **Aloe Vera (Aloe barbadensis miller):** • It cools and heals.

Uses: It calms sunburns, small burns, and skin irritations. Fresh aloe vera gel or products that you can buy are popular.

18. **Elderberry (Sambucus nigra):** Helps with the common cold and flu

Its properties are antiviral and immune-boosting.

Uses: Cuts down on the length of colds and flu. People often use elderberry syrup or pills.

19. **Garlic (Allium sativum):**

• It helps fight diseases and boosts the immune system. It works with either fresh garlic or garlic pills.

20. **(Echinacea purpurea):**

Properties: boosts the immune system and reduces inflammation.

Benefits: boosts the immune system and makes colds less severe. People often choose echinacea tincture or pills.

21. **Quercetin-Rich Herbs (e.g., Nettle, Quercetin supplements):**

Properties: Antihistaminic, anti-inflammatory.

Uses: Reduces allergy symptoms, such as sneezing and itching. Nettle tea or quercetin supplements are common.

22. **Butterbur (Petasites hybridus):**

Properties: Antihistaminic, anti-inflammatory.

Uses: Alleviates hay fever symptoms. Butterbur capsules are commonly used.

23. **Eyebright (Euphrasia officinalis):**

Properties: Anti-inflammatory, astringent.

Uses: Soothes irritated eyes and nasal passages. Eyebright tea or eyewash can be beneficial.

24. **Dong Quai (Angelica sinensis): Menstrual Discomfort:**

Properties: Uterine tonic, analgesic.

Uses: Regulates menstrual cycles, reduces cramps. Dong Quai capsules or tinctures are common.

25. Raspberry Leaf (Rubus idaeus):

Properties: Uterine tonic, astringent.

Uses: Supports female reproductive health, eases cramps. Raspberry leaf tea is commonly consumed.

26. Chaste Tree (Vitex agnus-castus):

Properties: Hormone-balancing, regulator.

Uses: Balances hormones, alleviates PMS symptoms. Chaste tree capsules or tinctures are commonly used.

27. Ginger (Zingiber officinale):

Properties: Anti-inflammatory, digestive.

Uses: Settles the stomach, aids digestion. Ginger tea or ginger capsules are effective options.

28. Marshmallow Root (Althaea officinalis):

Properties: Demulcent, soothing.

Uses: Eases irritation in the gastrointestinal tract. Marshmallow root tea or capsules can be helpful.

29. Cranberry (Vaccinium macrocarpon): Urinary Tract Infections (UTIs)

Properties: Antimicrobial, diuretic.

Uses: Prevents and supports the treatment of UTIs. Cranberry juice or capsules are commonly used.

30. Dandelion (Taraxacum officinale):

Properties: Diuretic, anti-inflammatory.

Uses: Supports kidney health and urinary function. Dandelion tea or capsules are effective.

31. Uva Ursi (Arctostaphylos uva-ursi):

Properties: Antimicrobial, astringent.

Uses: Assists in treating urinary tract infections. Uva ursi capsules or tinctures are common choices.

32. Hawthorn (Crataegus spp): High Blood Pressure

Properties: Cardiovascular tonic, vasodilator.

Uses: Supports heart health, helps regulate blood pressure. Hawthorn capsules or tinctures are popular.

33. Olive Leaf (Olea europaea):

Properties: Antihypertensive, antioxidant.

Uses: Assists in lowering blood pressure. Olive leaf extract or tea can be beneficial.

34. Ginkgo Biloba (Ginkgo biloba): Memory and Cognitive Function

Properties: Cognitive enhancer, antioxidant.

Uses: Improves memory and cognitive function. Ginkgo biloba capsules or extracts are commonly used.

35. Bacopa (Bacopa monnieri):

Properties: Nootropic, adaptogenic.

Uses: Enhances memory and cognitive performance. Bacopa capsules or tinctures are effective.

36. Rosemary (Rosmarinus officinalis):

Properties: Cognitive stimulant, antioxidant.

Uses: Improves focus and concentration. Rosemary essential oil or tea can be beneficial.

37. **Milk thistle (Silybum marianum**) has hepatoprotective and detoxifying properties.

Uses: Enhances liver function and detoxification. Milk thistle capsules and tinctures are popular.

38. **Arnica (Arnica montana) can** help with muscle soreness and inflammation.

Properties: anti-inflammatory and analgesic.

Uses: Reduces muscular discomfort and inflammation. Arnica gel and cream can be administered topically.

39. **Turmeric,** also known as Curcuma longa, has anti-inflammatory and analgesic properties.

Uses: Reduces inflammation and relieves muscle soreness. Turmeric pills and turmeric-infused meals are popular options.

40. Cayenne (Capsicum Annuum):

Properties: Analgesic and circulatory stimulant.

Used to relieve pain and promote circulation. Cayenne salves and creams can be used topically.

Chapter 16

Natural Herbs for all kinds of Disease

To be clear, natural therapies can help with some issues, but they shouldn't be relied upon in place of conventional medical care. In addition, the idea that a universal cure can treat "all kinds of diseases" is simplistic and ignores the complexity of human health. A personalized and evidence-based strategy is necessary for every health problem or disease.

 If you're looking for some natural remedies that may help your health, consider these 100 options. On the other hand, you should definitely talk to a doctor before adding them to your regimen:

Common Kitchen Ingredients

1. Turmeric: Anti-inflammatory and antioxidant properties.
2. Ginger: Anti-nausea and anti-inflammatory.
3. Garlic: Immune support and cardiovascular health.
4. Honey: Soothes sore throats and has antibacterial properties.
5. Lemon: Rich in vitamin C and aids digestion.
6. Apple Cider Vinegar: May help with digestion and blood sugar control.
7. Cinnamon: Anti-inflammatory and may help regulate blood sugar.
8. Chamomile: Calming, helps with sleep and digestive issues.
9. Peppermint: Relieves digestive discomfort and headaches.
10. Oregano: Contains antioxidants and has antimicrobial properties.
11. Basil: Anti-inflammatory and rich in antioxidants.
12. Rosemary: Improves digestion and cognitive function.
13. Thyme: Antimicrobial properties and immune support.
14. Sage: May support memory and cognitive function.

15. Lavender: Calming and may aid sleep.

16. Fennel: Eases digestive issues and supports heart health.

17. Licorice Root: Soothes the digestive tract and may help with respiratory issues.

18. Parsley: Rich in vitamins and may support kidney health.

19. Cayenne Pepper: Contains capsaicin with potential pain-relieving properties.

20. Cumin: Aids digestion and has anti-inflammatory effects.

Herbal Teas and Infusions

1. Green Tea: Rich in antioxidants and may support heart health.

2. Echinacea: Often used to support the immune system.

3. Nettle Tea: May help with allergies and inflammation.

4. Dandelion Tea: Supports liver health and digestion.

5. Lemon Balm Tea: Calming and aids digestion.

6. Ginseng Tea: Adaptogenic herb for stress support.

7. Peppermint Tea: Relieves digestive issues and headaches.

8. Chamomile Tea: Calming and supports sleep.

9. Ginger Tea: Anti-nausea and anti-inflammatory.

10. Turmeric Tea: Contains curcumin with anti-inflammatory properties.

11. Rosehip Tea: Rich in vitamin C and antioxidants.

12. Hibiscus Tea: Supports heart health and may lower blood pressure.

13. Valerian Root Tea: Promotes relaxation and aids sleep.

14. Passionflower Tea: Calming and may help with anxiety.

15. Fenugreek Tea: Supports digestion and lactation.

16. Mint Tea: Soothes digestive issues and freshens breath.

17. Thyme Tea: Contains antioxidants and may relieve respiratory issues.

18. Lemon Verbena Tea: Aids digestion and has a calming effect.

19. Sage Tea: May support memory and cognitive function.

20. Rooibos Tea: Rich in antioxidants and supports overall health.

Essential Oils

1. Lavender Essential Oil: Calming and promotes relaxation.
2. Peppermint Essential Oil: Relieves headaches and aids digestion.
3. Tea Tree Essential Oil: Antimicrobial and may support skin health.
4. Eucalyptus Essential Oil: Clears respiratory passages and supports the immune system.
5. Lemon Essential Oil: Energizing and may have antibacterial properties.
6. Chamomile Essential Oil: Calming and supports sleep.
7. Frankincense Essential Oil: Anti-inflammatory and may support immune health.
8. Rosemary Essential Oil: Improves concentration and supports respiratory health.
9. Ginger Essential Oil: Anti-nausea and may help with muscle pain..
10. Oregano Essential Oil: Antimicrobial and may support immune health.
11. Cinnamon Essential Oil: Anti-inflammatory and antioxidant.
12. Thyme Essential Oil: Antioxidant and supports respiratory health.
13. Bergamot Essential Oil: Uplifting and may have mood-enhancing effects.
14. Lemongrass Essential Oil: Refreshing and may have antimicrobial properties.
15. Clove Essential Oil: Antioxidant and anti-inflammatory.
16. Ylang Ylang Essential Oil: Calming and may help with stress and anxiety.
17. Patchouli Essential Oil: Grounding and may have anti-inflammatory effects.
18. Juniper Berry Essential Oil: Supports detoxification and has antioxidant properties.
19. Clary Sage Essential Oil: Hormone-balancing and may reduce stress.

Traditional Practices

1. Acupuncture: Traditional Chinese practice for pain relief and balance.
2. Ayurveda: Indian holistic system using herbs, diet, and lifestyle for balance.
3. Yoga: Combines physical postures, breath work, and meditation for holistic well-being.
4. Meditation: Mindfulness practice for stress reduction and mental well-being.
5. Tai Chi: Chinese martial art promoting balance, flexibility, and relaxation.

6. Reiki: Japanese energy healing technique for relaxation and stress reduction.

7. Traditional African Medicine: Uses indigenous plants for healing.

8. Traditional Native American Healing Practices: Herbal remedies, ceremonies, and rituals.

9. Traditional European Herbalism: Historical herbal practices from Europe.

10. Traditional Korean Medicine: Incorporates acupuncture, herbs, and holistic approaches.

11. Traditional Persian Medicine: Ancient system using natural remedies for health.

12. Traditional Tibetan Medicine: Balancing body and mind through natural methods.

13. Traditional Amazonian Medicine: Shamanic practices and herbal remedies.

14. Traditional Mexican Medicine: Heavily influenced by indigenous practices and herbs.

15. Traditional Japanese Kampo Medicine: Herbal remedies based on traditional Chinese medicine.

16. Traditional Unani Medicine: Ancient Greek-inspired system using natural remedies.

17. Traditional Egyptian Medicine: Ancient practices using herbs and rituals.

18. Traditional Roman Medicine: Influenced by Greek and Egyptian herbal traditions.

19. Traditional Islamic Medicine: Blends traditional practices with Islamic teachings.

20. Traditional Native Hawaiian Healing: Uses plants, spirituality, and rituals for health.

Miscellaneous Natural Approaches

1. Aromatherapy: Promotes mental and physical health through the application of aromatic chemicals.

2. The use of water for medicinal purposes is known as hydrotherapy.

3. Color Therapy: The practice of utilizing certain colors for the purpose of healing.

Fourth, herbal poultices, which include using herbs topically to treat a variety of conditions.

Connecting with the Earth through grounding or earthing may have positive effects on health.

Sixth, Taking a Dip in the River

Although natural remedies can be helpful for some health issues, it's important to remember that they shouldn't be used as a substitute for medical advice or treatment. In order to manage diseases in a thorough and individualized manner, it is essential to speak with a healthcare professional. When looking for a natural solution to a particular health problem, try these:

Chapter 17

Growing Your Herbal Garden

A sustainable and gratifying way to get fresh herbs for cooking, medicine, and aromatherapy is to grow your own herbal garden.

By following these steps, you can create a thriving herbal garden that provides you with fresh herbs for cooking, medicinal remedies, and aromatic pleasures throughout the year. Enjoy the process of nurturing your garden and exploring the many uses of your homegrown herbs!

- **Choose a Location**: Select a sunny spot in your garden that receives at least 6-8 hours of sunlight per day. Most herbs prefer well-drained soil, so make sure the area has good drainage.
- **Plan Your Garden**: Decide which herbs you want to grow based on your preferences and needs. Consider factors such as the climate in your area, the space available, and whether you want to focus on culinary herbs, medicinal herbs, or a combination of both.
- **Select Herbs**: Choose a variety of herbs that you enjoy cooking with or that have medicinal properties you can benefit from. Some popular culinary herbs to consider include basil, thyme, rosemary, parsley, mint, and oregano. For medicinal herbs, consider options like lavender, chamomile, echinacea, and lemon balm.
- **Start Seeds or Buy Seedlings**: Decide whether you want to start your herbs from seeds or purchase seedlings from a nursery or garden center. Starting from seeds allows you to have a wider selection of varieties, but it requires more time and attention. Seedlings provide a head start and are easier for beginners.
- **Prepare the Soil:** Prepare the soil by loosening it with a shovel or garden fork and removing any weeds or debris. Add compost or organic matter to improve soil fertility and structure.
- **Plant Herbs**: Plant your herbs according to their spacing requirements, which can vary depending on the plant. Some herbs, like mint, can be invasive and may need to be contained in pots or separate areas of the garden.

- **Water Regularly**: Keep your herbal garden well-watered, especially during dry periods. Most herbs prefer consistent moisture but can tolerate some drought once established.

- **Mulch:** Apply a layer of organic mulch, such as straw or wood chips, around your herbs to help retain moisture, suppress weeds, and regulate soil temperature.

- **Harvest Herbs**: Once your herbs have grown sufficiently, you can start harvesting them for culinary or medicinal use. Harvest herbs in the morning when the essential oils are most concentrated, and use sharp scissors or pruning shears to avoid damaging the plants.

- **Maintain Your Garden**: Regularly prune and deadhead your herbs to encourage bushy growth and prolong the harvest season. Keep an eye out for pests and diseases, and address any issues promptly using organic methods if possible.

Chapter 18

Tools and Equipment in Herbalism

Herbalism is the use of plants for medical and therapeutic reasons. To collect, prepare, and give herbal remedies, you often need specific tools and equipment. Here is a full list of the things that are usually used in herbalism:

1. **Pruning shears:** It cuts twigs, leaves, and flowers cleanly, which keeps plants healthy.
2. **Harvesting Knife:** • A sharp knife for cutting plant parts precisely. Great for getting roots and other parts that need to be cut cleanly.
3. **Herb scissors** are multi-bladed scissors that are made to cut herbs quickly and evenly. Works well for a lot of fresh herbs at once.
4. Gloves: • Keep your hands safe from thorns, irritants, and allergies.This is very helpful when working with plants that have spines or sap.

Tools for drying:

- ❖ Herb drying racks: • Hang herbs upside down to let them dry naturally in the air.Allows air to flow freely so that everything dries evenly.
- ❖ A dehydrator is an electric machine that lets you dry herbs quickly and precisely. Good for making a lot of things at once or in places with a lot of humidity.
- ❖ Muslin cloth or paper bags can be used to roll up and hang herbs to dry. Keeps herbs safe from dust and sunlight while they dry.

Processing and Grinding Tools:

Mortar and Pestle:

- Used for grinding herbs into powders or making herbal pastes.
- Allows for controlled crushing and grinding.

Herb Grinder:

- Electric or manual grinder for quickly processing larger quantities of herbs.
- Useful for making herbal blends, powders, or teas.

Food Processor or Blender:

- For making herbal extracts, smoothies, or incorporating herbs into various recipes.

Storage Containers:

Glass Jars:

- Ideal for storing dried herbs, tinctures, and infused oils.
- Avoids contamination and keeps herbs fresh.

Amber or Cobalt Glass Bottles:

- Best for storing liquid herbal extracts, tinctures, or infused oils.
- Protects contents from light, preserving their potency.

Airtight Containers:

- Ensures freshness by preventing air and moisture from reaching herbs.
- Useful for storing dried herbs or herbal preparations.

Measuring Tools:

Measuring Spoons and Cups:

- For precise measurement of dried herbs, powders, or liquid extracts.

Digital Scale:

- Useful for accurately weighing herbs when making formulations or tinctures.

Graduated Cylinders:

- For measuring and pouring liquid herbal preparations with precision.

Extraction Tools:

- Cheesecloth or Muslin Bags:
- Used for straining herbal infusions, decoctions, or tinctures.

Labeling Materials:

Labels and Markers:

- Essential for labeling jars, bottles, or storage containers with herb names, date, and preparation details.

Adhesive or Washable Labels:

- Ensures labels stay in place and remain legible despite exposure to moisture or handling.

Conclusion

These important plants promote natural and holistic health in your house. Try teas, tinctures, and infused oils to find the best way to use these herbs. Before taking herbs for medicine, visit a doctor or herbalist, especially if you are pregnant or have a health concern.

1. **Lavender (Lavandula angustifolia)** • Calming and Relaxing:

Lavender is known to relax. Use lavender essential oil in diffusers or sachets for a relaxing atmosphere. Use dried lavender in teas to relax and reduce tension.

• Skin Care

Lavender heals skin. Make lavender-infused oils or salves for mild burns, bug bites, and skin irritations. Many skin types can use its gentleness.

2. **Peppermint (Mentha × piperita) • Aids digestion**

For digestion, peppermint is recommended. Peppermint tea relieves indigestion, bloating, and nausea. Its pleasant taste complements food and drinks.

• Respiratory Health

Peppermint menthol helps respiratory health. Peppermint steam or tea can reduce congestion and calm the respiratory tract during colds and allergies.

3. **Chamomile (Matricaria chamomilla) • Relaxing Tea**

Chamomile tea is known for relaxing. To sleep, calm anxiety, and relax the nervous system, drink a cup before bed. The gentle choice is good for kids and adults.

• Skin soothing

Gentle chamomile is good for skin. Use chamomile in oils or creams to relieve eczema and mild rashes. Particularly useful for sensitive or irritated skin.

4. **Echinacea (Echinacea purpurea)** • immunological Support Echinacea is a powerful herb for immunological support. Make echinacea tinctures or teas to enhance immunity and shorten colds and flu. In winter, it's essential.

• Wound Healing

Echinacea's antibacterial qualities stimulate wound healing. Make salves or poultices for cuts, scrapes, and mild infections.

5. **Rosemary (Rosmarinus officinalis)**

• Delicious food

With its scent, rosemary enhances gourmet dishes. Try it in roasts, marinades, or infused oils for a herbal explosion. Due of its antioxidant properties, food is healthier.

• Cognitive Support

Rosemary improves mood. Inhale rosemary-infused steam or light a rosemary diffuser to boost focus, memory, and cognition.

6. **Aloe Vera (Aloe barbadensis)** • Skin Healing

Aloe vera is versatile in skin care. Aloe vera gel from a freshly broken leaf soothes sunburns, minor burns, and skin irritations. It soothes several skin conditions.

Digestive Aid

Digestion can benefit from aloe vera. Mix aloe vera gel into smoothies or drinks to help digestion and ease indigestion or acid reflux.

7. **Ginger (Zingiber officinale)**

• Digestive Comfort

Ginger is renowned for its digestive benefits. Brew ginger tea or incorporate fresh ginger into meals to alleviate nausea, indigestion, and promote overall digestive comfort.

• Anti-Inflammatory

Ginger possesses anti-inflammatory properties. Use fresh ginger in cooking or brew ginger tea to reduce inflammation, ease joint pain, and support overall joint health.

8. Thyme

Thyme is a powerful herb for respiratory health. Infuse thyme into teas or use it in culinary dishes to alleviate coughs, bronchitis, and congestion. Its antimicrobial properties contribute to overall immune support.

• Wound Antiseptic

Thyme's antibacterial properties treat wounds. Create thyme-infused oils or salves to cleanse and treat cuts, wounds, and skin infections.

9.Allium sativum garlic

• Immune Boost

Herb garlic boosts immunity. Eat raw garlic or use garlic supplements to boost immunity and fight colds and illnesses.

Garlic aids heart health. Garlic may reduce blood pressure, cholesterol, and heart disease.

10 .Calendula (officinalis)

Healing of the Skin

A soothing herb, calendula promotes skin healing. For faster wound healing, softer dry skin, and relief from eczema and dermatitis, try infusing calendula into an oil, cream, or salve.

Topical analgesics

Even when taken internally, calendula has anti-inflammatory effects. If you want to help your digestive system and lessen inflammation there, make some calendula tea.

11. **Curcuma longa**, or turmeric, has anti-inflammatory properties.

One plant that can effectively reduce inflammation is turmeric. Curries, drinks, or supplements made with turmeric can help with inflammation, joint health, and discomfort.

The Power of Antioxidants

It is a great supplement to your regular routine because of its antioxidant qualities. Optimal cellular health and resistance to oxidative stress may result from regular ingestion.

12. Calming Tea • Lemon Balm (Melissa officinalis)

Many people find that lemon balm helps them relax. In order to help you unwind, reduce tension, and get a good night's sleep, try brewing some lemon balm tea. This choice is mild enough for both children and adults to use.

References

Ody, P. (1993). The Complete Medicinal Herbal. Dorling Kindersley.

Tilgner, S. (1999). Herbal Medicine From the Heart of the Earth. Wise Acres LLC.

Green, J. (2000). The Herbal Medicine-Maker's Handbook. Crossing Press.

Pitchford, P. (2002). Healing with Whole Foods: Asian Traditions and Modern Nutrition. North Atlantic Books.

Murray, M. T., & Pizzorno, J. (2012). The Encyclopedia of Natural Medicine. Atria Books.

Elpel, T. J. (2004). Botany in a Day: The Patterns Method of Plant Identification. HOPS Press.

Newcomb, L. (1977). Newcomb's Wildflower Guide. Little, Brown and Company.

Martin, D. L. (2014). Rodale's Basic Organic Gardening. Rodale Books.

Lloyd, C. (1983). The Well-Tempered Garden. Frances Lincoln.

Storl, W. D. (1999). The Herbal Lore of Wise Women and Wortcunners. North Atlantic Books.

Buhner, S. H. (2002). The Lost Language of Plants: The Ecological Importance of Plant Medicines to Life on Earth. Chelsea Green Publishing.

Ody, P. (1993). The Complete Medicinal Herbal. Dorling Kindersley.

Tilgner, S. (1999). Herbal Medicine From the Heart of the Earth. Wise Acres LLC.

Green, J. (2000). The Herbal Medicine-Maker's Handbook. Crossing Press.

Pitchford, P. (2002). Healing with Whole Foods: Asian Traditions and Modern Nutrition. North Atlantic Books.

Murray, M. T., & Pizzorno, J. (2012). The Encyclopedia of Natural Medicine. Atria Books.

Elpel, T. J. (2004). Botany in a Day: The Patterns Method of Plant Identification. HOPS Press.

Newcomb, L. (1977). Newcomb's Wildflower Guide. Little, Brown and Company.

Martin, D. L. (2014). Rodale's Basic Organic Gardening. Rodale Books.

Lloyd, C. (1983). The Well-Tempered Garden. Frances Lincoln.

Storl, W. D. (1999). The Herbal Lore of Wise Women and Wortcunners. North Atlantic Books.

Buhner, S. H. (2002). The Lost Language of Plants: The Ecological Importance of Plant Medicines to Life on Earth. Chelsea Green Publishing.